The Departme

'This intensive research is the definitive detailed proof of how government austerity hasn't just harmed disabled people, it has killed them. What is shocking is that government ministers knew the brutality of the system was causing such a loss of life and did nothing. John Pring's exposé of this killer system forms the charge sheet against the policy makers who inflicted this inhumane system on the most vulnerable in our society.'

—John McDonnell MP

'A must-read exposé of one of Britain's biggest hidden scandals. Every politician, civil servant and journalist in the country should have this on their bookshelf.'

—Frances Ryan, *Guardian* journalist and author of *Crippled: Austerity and the Demonisation of Disabled People*

'John Pring's indefatigable research has revealed how successive Conservative, Labour and Coalition governments have not only failed to provide the money, help, resources and understanding that disabled people need, they have gone to great lengths to hide the truth about what they have done. It would be a strong person who could read this disturbing book in a sitting. But it must be read.'

—Paul Lewis, freelance financial journalist and presenter of *Money Box*, BBC Radio 4

'*The Department* is an expertly crafted, vigorously researched response to the gas-lighting endured by disabled benefit claimants at the hands of government and the DWP for the past 14 years. Pring, a journalist who is regarded within the disability community as a modern-day hero for his relentless pursuit of truth and justice, sensitively describes the terrible human cost of a social security system turned violent bureaucracy and gives voices to its victims. In also exposing the key players and decisions involved in causing and concealing mass harm, this book is a powerful call to arms for all decent human beings.'

—Ellen Clifford, author of *The War on Disabled People: Capitalism, Welfare and the Making of a Human Catastrophe*

'Like a dark whodunnit, where a government department is the killer, John Pring's *The Department* is a vital must-read book. Written by someone who has played a central role in uncovering how welfare reform kills disabled people, *The Department* comes out of over a decade of painstaking research and interviews with families whose loved ones have died. Pring heartbreakingly shows how policy signed off in Whitehall can end someone's life miles away in distance and time. The book is an essential history and a call for action and solidarity right now.'

—China Mills, Disability Justice Lead, Healing Justice London

'No other journalist has done as much over the past 14 years to shed light on the multiple injustices directed at disabled people in the UK as a result of austerity and so-called "welfare reform". John's book is a "must read" for anyone who seeks the truth.'

—Mary O'Hara, author of *Austerity Bites: A Journey to the Sharp End of Cuts in the UK*

'An urgent book that tells of the injustice, hostility and violence levelled at disabled people, by government departments responsible for their welfare. The scapegoating and stigma orchestrated by Conservative and Labour governments from the 1990s up to the current austerity reforms is shocking, and Pring's accounts of those most affected will leave you feeling sad and enraged. This book is a long time coming and will have enormous relevance for years to come, as governments try to enforce more budgetary cuts with the same ideological hostility levelled at disabled people.'

—Victoria Cooper, co-editor of *The Violence of Austerity*

The Department

How a Violent Government Bureaucracy Killed Hundreds and Hid the Evidence

John Pring

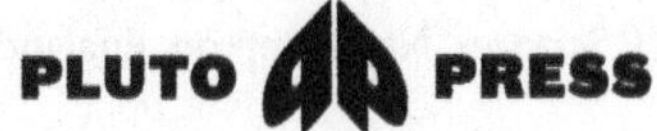

First published 2024 by Pluto Press
New Wing, Somerset House, Strand, London WC2R 1LA
and Pluto Press, Inc.
1930 Village Center Circle, 3-834, Las Vegas, NV 89134

www.plutobooks.com

British Library Cataloguing in Publication Data
A catalogue record for this book is available from the British Library

ISBN 978 0 7453 4989 3 Paperback
ISBN 978 0 7453 4991 6 PDF
ISBN 978 0 7453 4990 9 EPUB

This book is printed on paper suitable for recycling and made from fully managed and sustained forest sources. Logging, pulping and manufacturing processes are expected to conform to the environmental standards of the country of origin.

Typeset by Stanford DTP Services, Northampton, England

Simultaneously printed in the United Kingdom and United States of America

By slow violence I mean a violence that occurs gradually and out of sight, a violence of delayed destruction that is dispersed across time and space, an attritional violence that is typically not viewed as violence at all.

– Rob Nixon, *Slow Violence and the Environmentalism of the Poor*, 2013

Time is key to understanding the everyday, bureaucratic, and institutional violence of welfare reform, and how this violence kills people.

– Dr China Mills, 2023

Contents

PART III
2010–14: The Coalition, Austerity, and Deaths by Welfare

PART IV
2014–22: Cover-up, Investigations, and the Truth about DWP

Preface

'Hundreds of deaths!?' he cries.

On the other end of the line is Professor Sir Mansel Aylward, architect of the 'all work test', introduced in 1995 by the Department of Social Security (DSS) to assess whether disabled people were eligible for out-of-work disability benefits or, instead, were 'fit for work'. Now 80 years old, he is still working two days a week at Cardiff University. I hope our conversation will be the final piece in a grim puzzle that stretches across five decades.

I have just told him how academics concluded that the introduction of a new assessment process in 2008 – built on the structure he devised in the early 1990s – was linked to nearly 600 suicides over just three years in the early 2010s.

'The figures you quote to me are, you know, I just don't understand. Something's gone wrong,' he says. He insists there were no such large-scale deaths when the all work test was introduced. 'Why is it happening now?' he asks.

This is the complex and disturbing question *The Department* seeks to answer. To do this, it examines the bureaucratic violence inflicted on disabled people who have relied on the benefits system since the late 1980s. As my friend and collaborator Dr China Mills – who introduced me to the idea of slow bureaucratic violence – says, the consideration of time is crucial to understanding how this happened; how the everyday actions of bureaucrats, ministers and private sector executives combined to inflict awful violence on disabled people who rely on the welfare state. But just as this violence has been slow, so has the process of uncovering its course. This book is the result of more than a decade of research and reporting and, most importantly, listening to disabled people and grieving relatives.

I was not the first to draw links between the actions of the Department for Work and Pensions (the successor to the DSS) – and its ministers, civil servants, and private sector contractors – and the deaths of disabled people who relied on the social security safety net. I have drawn heavily on other people's work, particularly research carried out by the disabled people's movement. Without that work, this book would have been impossible.

My own obsessive search for information about these deaths has filled in gaps and found answers to deeply troubling questions that began to emerge in the austerity years of the 2010 coalition government. At first, I used the Freedom of Information Act, and more recently I have been trawling through the National Archives to find government memos and letters from the 1990s and early 2000s that help explain the shocking events I will describe in the following pages.

I also felt a need to tell the stories of those who died, through the recollections of family members and – where possible – through their own words, and documents they left behind. As a disabled person myself, with lifelong suicidal ideation and a recent autism diagnosis, I recognise my need for these innocent victims of government hostility to be remembered, and for justice to be secured.

The deaths I describe in *The Department* are only a tiny fraction of those that could be linked to the actions of the Department for Work and Pensions, known by most benefit claimants as the DWP. Most of these deaths will remain hidden, particularly if those who died did not have family or friends to fight for justice in their names. I hope the disabled people I do write about can represent all those who lost their lives through this terrible, violent episode, and those who continue to do so.

In keeping with the theme of slow violence, the book is structured chronologically. It begins with an examination of how John Major's Conservative government first targeted – and scapegoated – disabled benefit claimants as 'a promising area for making economies', and how these reforms slowly began to have a deadly impact. In this section, particularly, I hope my research in the National Archives has produced some fascinating and disturbing revelations.

Part II looks at the New Labour years of 1997 to 2010, and how the party's significant change in tone on welfare reform after Tony

Blair's election as Labour leader eventually had a fatal impact on the disability benefits system. These are also the years when the private sector tightened its grip on the system. Again, with deadly effect.

Part III describes how the reckless hostility and discrimination that had built slowly over the previous two decades finally exploded into deadly violence in the early years of the coalition, from 2010 onwards. It was disabled activists who produced the research that first exposed this harm, describing the deep distress, the self-harm, and the suicide attempts – a 'climate of panic' – that should have persuaded the government to act, but didn't. As austerity intensified, a series of tragedies showed how this violence devastated the lives of disabled people across boundaries of race, sex, and class.

In the final section, I show how DWP attempted to cover up and justify its actions, as it had to a lesser extent in the previous two decades, and angrily resisted appeals from disabled people and their allies to make the system safe. Despite these efforts at cover-up and denial, evidence of negligence, dishonesty and hostility slowly emerged, through coroners' reports, the department's own secret reviews, and the courage and determination of those left behind. What is revealed, I hope, is the truth about DWP, and a clear and powerful demand for change and – finally – justice.

Content Advice

You're likely to come to this book with some idea of its content, and an awareness that much of it will be distressing and disturbing. It contains repeated discussion of suicide and other deaths, and descriptions of people in significant mental and physical distress. To help with this, at the end of this book there is an index of pages that could be particularly triggering. Please only read *The Department* when you feel ready. Also, reading something distressing can sometimes affect us not just immediately but in the days or even weeks to come. If you think this could apply to you, you might wish to limit how much you read in one sitting, to reduce any unexpected future impact. I believe the information revealed in this book is valuable, but your safety is more important.

Introduction: The Death of Philippa Day

2019

I'm not dying because I'm suicidal and that sounds ridiculous. It's pragmatic. Yes a dead mum and a shit father will hurt my child for the rest of his life but that's better than watching mummy go in and out of hospital, crying everyday being triggered everyday … I dragged myself up from the bottom basically every 24 hours for just over 27 years … I've been so trapped for so long and then comes along the government people would assume are there to help. Since January the 11th 2019 my benefits have been severely cut, this has caused me to get pay day loans to simply live and that has escalated into a hole I can never get out of … having nothing has isolated me even more from the world, has affected my identity. I haven't had a haircut for over a year for fucks sake.

This time feels different. I'm scared … Please protect [my son] from this awful world … There is hope for [his] future, that's Imogen Day. She's gonna change the world. Thank fuck for that.

My name is Philippa Day I'm a good person, I'm strong as fuck. I'm a damn good mother when I had the opportunity … Tess I'm sorry. I tried I really did.

This is all pointless I don't even know why I'm writing this, like it matters.

I'm sorry.

Peace Out

*12.02.92 – 08.08.19**

* As Philippa was dyslexic, parts of this letter have been edited to make it more readable and accessible.

Imogen Day has the clearest memories of her sister, Pip (or Philippa, as the DWP knew her). She was eight and Pip was four years older and would hide Imogen's treasured teddy bear. 'It was her favourite activity to make me go hunting round the house, just to watch me tear the house apart. She thought it was hilarious. She would give me clues but would never allow it to go on too long, so when I got too upset she would stop ...'

Pip would defend her sister at school if she was bullied. 'She was the only one who was allowed to tease me,' Imogen would tell me. Their parents both worked, so the girls attended an after-school club. Pip would arrange Imogen's toys around her and put her sister on her lap until they were picked up.

'So many things brought her joy,' Imogen would tell the Deaths by Welfare podcast. 'She was a really, really happy, kind person. She loved her friends; she loved just engaging with different people. She was always the first person to give a homeless person a cigarette, and would sit and chat with them. She had so much empathy for the world.'

Her mum, Jane, says Pip was 'full of love and kindness', and used to 'bounce into rooms; everyone knew that she'd come to the party'.

Both Pip's type one diabetes and her mental distress had been a part of her life for as long as Imogen could remember. Her parents had taken her as a child to courses to help her manage her diabetes. Pip would carry her needles and test kit in her handbag. She would slip away to the bathroom without any fuss. She was dyslexic and adapted to that, too.

Her mental health was different. She ran away from home and would show 'extreme emotions'. For a while, she was in foster care. There was a spell in a mental health unit. She used her insulin to self-harm, by failing to pay attention to her medication regime, by deliberately mismanaging her diet, or by overdosing.

At 17, Pip moves into her own flat, supported by her parents. She is diagnosed with bipolar disorder; later, the diagnosis changes to emotionally unstable personality disorder. She has difficulties maintaining personal relationships, anxiety, regulating her emotions, increasing problems with substance abuse, self-harm, and suicidal ideation. She places herself in situations where she is intensely vulnerable to harm.

By her early 20s, Pip has found a customer services job. She is using drugs recreationally, mostly cannabis and occasionally cocaine, and alcohol if with friends, although she will always check the sugar content. Her friends look out for her. But she is also in a toxic relationship.

Pip has a son in 2015 [a court order means he cannot be named], but experiences post-natal depression, and splits up with the father just after their son's first birthday. There is a 'non-molestation' court order and her ex's behaviour leads Pip to develop agoraphobia. She experiences physical, psychological, and sexual abuse from her ex, who frequently exploits her mental distress.

Pip's parents often take their grandson for a few days, sometimes at short notice if she is struggling. She is desperate to protect her son, to ensure he has a loving family around him.

By 2017, Pip and her family have decided her parents should look after her son semi-permanently. They live nearby, about 20 minutes by car, but she struggles with the idea that she cannot care for her son. This is exploited by her ex-partner. His abuse is later described by a safeguarding review as 'unremitting'. He strikes her head with a glass jar, and receives an 18-month community sentence. He repeatedly breaches a non-molestation order, and continues to exploit her mental distress. Eventually he is sentenced to 20 weeks in prison, but immediately contacts Pip on his release. The harassment and stalking continue.

Pip tells a domestic violence adviser: 'He took the city I grew up in and made it a place I couldn't stand to be anymore.' And, after a court has extended a suspended sentence following another breach: 'That's what broke me. I report and do everything and then nothing happens. These orders are not worth the paper they are written on.'

Pip is now living in a pretty, red-brick house – owned by her parents – on a residential road of manicured gardens and unvarnished picket fences, north-east of the centre of Nottingham. Her dad keeps the front door key for emergencies. Pip uses the kitchen door, set back from the front of the house. On the tarmac driveway, and the wall, there are often pastel chalk pictures Pip has drawn for her son. There is a rainbow one week, a tiger the next. She persuades her son to practice writing his name on the wall.

Life is 'a rollercoaster' for the family, says Imogen. Pip once told her she felt like an electric wire, stripped of its protective rubber coating. Touching the wire creates sparks of anxiety, depression, and hopelessness. Or alternatively, extreme positivity, love, and elation. Everything is extreme, including her feelings about other people. 'You were a hero or a villain,' says Imogen.

Pip's drug use is increasing. She has told Imogen about her thoughts of self-harm and suicide. Imogen talks to her about her drug use. As it increases, Pip falls out with her friends. She begins to rely increasingly on her family, particularly her father and sister.

In March 2018, Pip is allocated a care coordinator, community psychiatric nurse (CPN) Tessa Rand, following a period under the mental health crisis team. There had been an overdose in autumn 2017 – the second of that year – and a spell in hospital. Tessa, who will become a trusted, invaluable part of Pip's life, will later tell an inquest that Pip felt stigmatised by the personality disorder diagnosis. 'She felt she was judged as acting out to get attention. That bothered her a lot because this was Philippa's way of communicating her distress.'

Pip tells Tessa she should be able to look after her own son. 'It saddened her deeply that she couldn't do that,' said Tessa. 'It also made her angry with herself and others that she felt had let her down.'

Pip's ex is causing her 'an incredible amount of stress'. Pip struggles with the idea that she might see him, or his friends, or he might be following her. 'As time went on, it translated into struggling to go out at all,' Tessa will say later. 'In the last few months, she couldn't go out alone.'

Suicidal thoughts are ever-present, and thoughts of self-harm will turn to action when the thoughts become particularly intense. She cuts and burns herself. There are at least five overdoses in 2018. Tessa believes Pip is 'incredibly knowledgeable' about how much insulin she can take without killing herself. There are times when there is plenty left after an overdose.

In late 2018, Pip is advised to apply for personal independence payment (PIP). She had been given a lifetime award of disability living allowance in 1994 (at the middle rate of care) because of her diabetes – this entitled her to disability premiums on top of income support – but she is told she will probably receive more with PIP. She phones DWP for a claim form. Imogen accompanies her to an advice agency that helps her fill out the form.

Tessa writes a letter to support her claim, and makes it clear Pip will need to be assessed at home. Tessa remembers driving with Pip in January 2019 when she asks her to pull over so she can post her PIP form. 'We made a huge deal of her achieving this task, which would be small for many but enormous for Pip,' says Imogen.

Pip starts mentalisation-based therapy, which seems to help her examine her life in a new way. It is one of many ways she engages with services in her last years. Her agoraphobia and distrust of professionals mean nearly every engagement is difficult, but she attends appointments, engages with Tessa and her colleagues, takes medication, liaises with her GP, speaks with a psychiatrist and clinical psychologist, spends time as an inpatient and, eventually, takes steps towards engaging with substance misuse services.

By February 2018, Pip realises she is short of money. She doesn't know why and blames herself. The reason soon becomes clear. DWP has closed both her new PIP claim and her existing DLA claim, while also reducing her income support, and cutting her payments by a further £12.43 to repay a previous Social Fund loan. Her weekly benefits plummet from £228.25 to just £63.10. DWP had sent her a letter on 11 January explaining that she had failed to return her PIP form, so her DLA claim would end on 29 January. She never opened the letter. Pip has been receiving DLA since she was 16, a lifetime award.

'I would often go to her house and find letters that were weeks old that had not been opened,' said her father, Charles, later. 'She never knew what was going to be in the letter and therefore was fearful of the letter.'

Tessa calls DWP and says Pip had been unwell. The department promises to look for the missing form. There is no evidence this search ever took place. Pip is distraught. On 19 March, she self-harms by cutting and burning herself, and takes excessive medication with alcohol. Her ex's harassment continues. It is, the safeguarding review will say later, 'insidious'. At one point he deposits 10p into her bank account so he can add a reference about himself, which 'signalled that he was still there, still controlling her'.

The following day, DWP looks again at the decision to close her claims, but – despite Tessa's call – leaves it unchanged. It also fails to mark on its system that Pip needs 'additional support'.

Pip is admitted to a mental health unit. On 1 April, she takes another insulin overdose, after alerting a friend through Facebook. 'There wasn't a time when I worked with her that she took a significant overdose without letting somebody know,' Tessa told the inquest later.

On 4 April, Philippa begins a fresh PIP claim. She is discharged from hospital for bringing cocaine onto the ward. Her family are distraught, because it is a specialist personality disorder unit and they thought she would receive the support she needed.

The downward spiral continues. Pip begins acting out of character. She smashes a car window after hallucinating that a man inside the car is trying to kill her. She is admitted to another psychiatric hospital. Pip asks Imogen during a visit if she will fight for her after she dies, to ensure others are not 'left to die' by DWP. She has read about disabled people in similar situations who have lost their lives due to austerity. 'They are trying to fucking kill me,' she tells her sister. Pip leaves the hospital after just a few days, partly because the staff will not allow her to control her diabetes herself. It is one of the few things she feels she can control.

The gaps between overdoses grow shorter, although she will always alert a friend or her father and leave the front door unlocked. Pip tells her sister she is stuck, she has no money, and has taken out payday loans with huge interest rates.

Almost every day, Pip talks to Imogen about her PIP application. She feels worthless. The process is dragging on, and although her family and Tessa are trying to support her, her drug use is increasing, and, for the first time, she begins taking drugs on her own. During one visit, Pip asks Tessa to open a bin bag and she dumps a pile of unopened correspondence straight into it.

Tessa writes another supportive letter, describing the two recent hospital admissions, and her financial worries. Her diabetes nurse also writes a letter. Pip completes the new claim form, and her father posts it to DWP by recorded delivery.

Pip is now surviving on £60 a week. She doesn't shower or bath regularly because she hates seeing her own body. She takes less care of the house. She starts talking more about suicide.

On 11 June, growing ever desperate, Pip phones DWP. The call is recorded. 'Basically I need to find out the progress of my claim,' says Pip. 'It's been six months now and I'm literally starving and cold.' There is little empathy from Jane, the DWP telephone agent, who says her form has been sent to Capita. 'You're better to ring them and see what their plans are,' she says. She tells her to visit her local 'jobs and benefits office' about money.

Pip's voice is breaking with distress. 'I shouldn't have had this taken away from me. My DLA was for my type one diabetes, which is not curable and lifelong. This is six months. I'm in so much debt.' Her voice breaks again. 'I haven't had anything to eat. I can't …' Her words tail away into quiet sobs.

After a moment or two, Pip says she will ring Capita, and asks the DWP worker to log the call.

'Yeah, it'll be on the system,' she is told.

'Thank you. Sorry.'

'Is that everything I can help you with?'

'Well no, not really. I need a [unclear]. I need a reason to live. Thank you. Goodbye.'

'Would you be able to apply for the ESA?'

'I'm on income support.' Her voice quivers. 'All of my disability premiums have been taken away from me because of this damn PIP form. I should have never, ever, ever have been transferred over from DLA to PIP. This has been six months long, I'm in £5,000 worth of debt. I'm …'

'Is there anybody in your family or a local charity that could help you out?'

'No, no there isn't, because I ...' her voice breaks again. She sobs. 'If this isn't solved quickly then, I, I ...' and suddenly the sobbing stops and there is clarity, '... I cannot survive, physically survive, for another eight weeks, six weeks, four weeks, whatever, without any money ... So yeah, alright, I'll call the other people.' The call ends.

Jane will later tell an inquest Pip appeared 'content' at the end of the call. She says it is 'quite usual' to hear claimants crying and can't remember why she failed to leave a summary note on Pip's file. She also can't remember why she hadn't discussed the call with a manager. And she is unsure if she passed any information to Capita.

Two days later, Tessa visits Pip. 'She didn't seem to be looking after herself very well,' Tessa told the inquest. 'She told me she didn't have any food in the fridge. I was quite concerned, because of her type one diabetes.'

Between 12 and 18 June, Tessa calls DWP six times. She says Pip is £5,000 in debt and has no food or heating, and had not been opening her post in January. As a result, Pip's DLA is finally reinstated on 18 June and DWP sends her £1,160 as partial payment of her arrears, which is immediately swallowed up by her debts. But DWP and Capita must still process her new PIP claim. Pip tells Imogen she believes she will be dead before this happens.

Tessa visits Pip. She notes her chaotic home life and escalating drug use. Pip tells Tessa she is in considerable debt to drug-dealers.

On 20 June, another £869 in arrears is paid into Pip's bank account after part of her disability premium is reinstated. On 26 June, Capita decides she must have a face-to-face assessment.

Pip's alcohol and drug misuse worsens. Those visiting her home are heavier drug users than her previous friends.

Pip speaks to Tessa of her shame that she can't be part of her son going to his new school in September. 'She started to feel she had lost her son,' said Tessa. 'She had always counted her son as a strong protective force, but she was doing so less often by that time.' On 2 July, Pip's parents and her son go abroad on holiday. They need a break, and Pip is too unwell to join them. Three days later, Pip writes a letter on her laptop.

Letter to Dad upon death
Well, where the fuck do I start? I guess an apology but I think if everyone was honest with themselves me no longer being around causes less problems than me being alive.

Any other father would have given up a long time, so thank you and sorry your faith was misplaced … My fondest memories along with [my son's] life, was going to work with you on a Saturday, I'd feel so important … I remember you kissing my forehead after [my son] was born …

They say play the cards you're dealt, but that would also mean bowing out when you have no hope of a full house. I never was very good at poker, or life really. Hindsight really is useless isn't it.

I refuse to prolong my son's pain in hoping I'll get better. 3 years later I'm still broken, possibly more so.

I know you never read this shit. I just wanted to say I'm sorry. Always have been the weak link in the family.

*Philippa**

On 16 July, Pip is told by Capita she will need to attend a face-to-face assessment at a centre in Nottingham on 1 August. The idea terrifies her. She becomes angrier, and more depressed, and considers cancelling her claim. It later emerges that Capita has heard about Pip's self-harm and is concerned about the risk of 'weapons' in her house, and so rules out a home assessment. It could have checked with her mental health team, but doesn't.

Imogen, who has been supporting Pip, returns home to Leeds to finish her dissertation. She tries to reassure her they will secure a home assessment, but Pip has lost all faith in DWP and Capita.

On 31 July, one of Tessa's colleagues visits Pip. She phones Capita to discuss the assessment, due to take place the next day. She

* As Philippa was dyslexic, parts of this letter have been edited to make it more readable and accessible.

explains Pip's level of distress and asks yet again for a home assessment, explaining her agoraphobia. She is told to provide written evidence. The assessment is postponed until 19 August to allow time to provide that evidence.

Pip receives another letter, confirming she will need to attend the face-to-face assessment on 19 August. The letter says it is 'important to go to this appointment', otherwise DWP is 'likely to refuse your claim'.

On 7 August, Imogen hears Pip's home assessment request has been rejected. 'I felt such a dread when I heard this,' says Imogen. 'She would have sobbed, she would have screamed, she would have experienced immense distress and frustration and would have been unable to communicate [if she had been forced to visit a Capita assessment centre]. I would have been very concerned about an overdose directly after the assessment.'

Pip calls Tessa. 'I'm done,' she tells her. 'I can't do this anymore, I can't cope.'

Tessa phones Capita twice. All they will see is how distressed Pip is, she says. Capita asks her to provide written evidence but cannot explain what else they need. DWP later admits Tessa's phone call should have been enough. Tessa calls Pip again but can't get through. She speaks to Pip's father, who says he will join her at the assessment. Tessa calls Capita again to say Pip will attend the face-to-face assessment if she can accompany her.

Charles Day speaks to his daughter twice on 7 August, the first time to tell Pip she will have to attend the assessment centre. 'I think that was the final straw,' he will say later.

Pip knew her family would never abandon her. 'It's the only thing she knew for certain,' he says. Her family shop for her, and cook and deliver meals, but asking for money from her dad would 'massively' damage her sense of self-worth. He speaks to Pip later. She will usually ask to say goodnight to her son, but this time she doesn't want to. They arrange to speak the following afternoon.

When Imogen speaks to her sister, she can tell Pip is having a panic attack. She calms her down with some breathing exercises and tries to reassure her about a home assessment. But Pip tells her: 'I'm done trying to fight them.'

Imogen asks to meet for lunch the next day, a safeguarding technique as Pip often speaks of how devastated she will be if Imogen or their father find her after a suicide attempt. But Pip says she has an appointment, and they agree to meet on the ninth. Imogen reassures her that they will find a solution. They continue to exchange messages through the evening. Imogen will say later: 'We were just having very casual sisterly conversations about our daily lives.' Then, just after midnight, Pip stops responding. Imogen assumes she has fallen asleep.

The next day, Imogen and Charles become increasingly concerned when they cannot contact Pip. When they arrive at her house, they find it 'in its usual disarray'.

Upstairs, Imogen finds Pip lying with her limbs strewn across her bed. On one corner of the bed, by her bleeding head, is the letter from Capita telling her the request for a home assessment has been rejected.

PART I

1989–97
Peter Lilley, Incapacity Benefit, and How Ill-health Became a Luxury

1
The First Memo

Where should this story begin? With the introduction of invalidity benefit in 1971? The creation of the modern welfare state in 1948? Perhaps the Liberals' welfare reforms of the early 1900s, or the Elizabethan Poor Laws of 1598 and 1601, which required all parishes to provide a minimum level of support for those in need. Maybe it should begin with the Poor Law Amendment Act of 1834, which was based on the principle that life for those relying on state welfare should be unpleasant ... and should be seen by potential claimants to be unpleasant.

Even so, from the start of the twentieth century, through the development of Labour's post-war welfare state, and until the 1980s, there was a gradual move towards providing all citizens with security from 'the cradle to the grave'. But during the 1980s, this principle came under attack from Margaret Thatcher's Conservative government, and attention eventually turned to disabled people.

It is here, then, that this story begins, as civil servants, politicians, and the private sector start to question how they can pick away at the threads of the safety net.

Early in 1989, secretary of state for social security John Moore sends a memo to John Major, chief secretary to the Treasury.[1]

> ... I think it would be sensible to discuss the general approach to disability benefits.
>
> Both of us have acknowledged the need to tackle the rising expenditure on these benefits, but also that we can hardly ignore the [Office of Population Censuses and Surveys] disability surveys. I enclose a paper which presents our conclusions about how to handle this, with a package of proposals hewn from a

> mass of work over the last year or so. Politically, the context in which the surveys were commissioned and the results they now provide leave us no choice but to put forward a package offering long-term savings tempered by some benefit improvements in the interim …
>
> For me, the key issue is not whether we adopt a package such as proposed in the attached paper, but when …

Moore would be replaced as social security secretary months later by Tony Newton. John Major would become prime minister the following year. But the memo sets successive governments on a path that will lead to the deaths of hundreds, and probably thousands, of disabled people.

In 1989, the payment for those unable to work through ill-health or disability is known as invalidity benefit, which was introduced in 1971. The claimant's GP plays a significant role. They provide the 'sick note', describing their patient's 'incapacity for work'. For the first six months, the GP needs to consider their incapacity in relation to their usual occupation; if they had been a miner, are they able to work as a miner? But after six months on statutory sick pay or sickness benefit, the GP must decide if they are also unfit for other work and therefore eligible for the longer-term invalidity benefit (IVB).[2]

The Department of Social Security (DSS) supervises IVB claims. Claims are decided by adjudication officers in local DSS offices, which can refer claims to the Regional Medical Service (RMS) for an 'alternative medical opinion', mostly provided by retired or practising GPs.

If RMS decides there needs to be a medical examination, it will ask the GP for an up-to-date report, before carrying out the assessment. The DSS adjudication officer (AO) will then decide the claimant's eligibility 'in the light of all the available evidence', including the examination results. The RMS opinion is usually accepted. In 1991, about 600,000 claims are referred to RMS, with a third called for an examination. More than 80 per cent of claims referred to RMS are found 'incapable of work' and eligible for IVB.

Concerns about the growth in invalidity benefit spending lead the National Audit Office (NAO) to commission research from polling organisation Gallup.[3] The Gallup study finds serious problems, particularly with the lack of training and guidance for GPs on sick note work.

NAO publishes its report in January 1990. It says the number of IVB recipients has risen from 760,000 in 1983–84 to just over one million in 1987–88. DSS expects this to rise to 1.3 million by 1990–91, with spending expected to increase from £2.39 billion in 1983–84 to more than £4 billion in 1990–91 (at 1989 prices). The key reason is that individuals are staying on the benefit for longer, while the proportion of older IVB recipients is increasing, as is the number of married women receiving IVB. NAO concludes that these and other 'non-medical factors', including an increase in unemployment in the early 1980s, have probably played a 'significant part' in the increase.

The Gallup survey finds 32 per cent of GPs had not refused a single sick note request in six months. It concludes that many GPs are 'overlooking the requirement to consider the individual's capacity for alternative work' and 'giving too much weight to family and social circumstances'.

There is nothing to suggest widespread fraud, and yet the mainstream media leap on the survey results to attack disabled claimants and GPs. Press coverage on 12 January 1990 suggests DSS briefed the media to scapegoat claimants, with headlines including '£4bn row over "lead swinging"' (*The Sun*); 'Scandal of sick notes' (*Daily Mail*); and 'GPs' charter for workshy' (*Daily Express*). Even the liberal and left-wing media join in, with 'Soft GPs rapped' (*Daily Mirror*); 'Saving on sickness benefit urged' (*The Independent*); and '"Fit" jobless get sick benefit' (*The Guardian*).[4]

The report – particularly how it has been reported – provides vital political cover for DSS and its ministers to cut spending on IVB.

Months later, the Commons public accounts committee offers a more nuanced account of the NAO research, with its report[5] raising concerns about a possible backlash against disabled people.

It identifies three major trends, and none of them relate to 'soft GPs' or 'lead swinging'. Instead, claimants are staying on IVB for longer, there is a rising proportion of older recipients, and the number of married women receiving IVB is increasing. Other reasons include the lack of suitable alternative work for those no longer 'fit' for their previous occupation, while people are living longer because of advances in medicine. And, due to Care in the Community, where government policy had shifted away from institutional care and towards supporting disabled people, particularly those with mental distress or learning difficulties, in their own homes – more people are receiving invalidity benefit 'to which they were not entitled when in institutional care'.

The committee also raises an issue that will reappear in the austerity years of the 2010s, noting 'with concern the rise in the number and percentage of successful appeals in recent years by claimants who had been disallowed benefits', which could 'indicate an increasing degree of inequity' in the treatment of claims by adjudication officers. Between 1984 and 1988, the number of appeals had increased from about 2,000 to just under 4,000 a year, with the proportion of successful appeals rising from 34 to 50 per cent.

DSS is not particularly worried about losing 50 per cent of such cases, 'but would be concerned if this rose to 75 per cent' (which it will in 2019[6]). The committee says: 'The Department felt the figures did not support the view that they were harrying back to work large numbers of people who were incapable of work.'

By the end of 1990, the Treasury is agitating for savings, asking DSS for more details about the 'implementation of the £8 million saving' on invalidity benefit that has been agreed.[7] The pressure is slowly building.

2

A Promising Area for Cuts, and the First Steps towards Violence

April 1992. The Conservatives, under John Major, unexpectedly win the general election. Major appoints former trade secretary Peter Lilley as his secretary of state for social security, a post he will hold throughout the next five years.

Within weeks, Lilley meets fellow Thatcherite Michael Portillo, chief secretary to the Treasury. They pick on invalidity benefit as, in the words of a DSS civil servant,[1] 'one of the areas to be addressed in terms of the extent to which benefit arrangements match up to the circumstances of the 1990s'. A DSS memo[2] says Lilley 'has already indicated that he sees IVB as a promising area for making economies and has asked us to give more thought to what might be done to achieve this'.

A draft invalidity benefit (IVB) policy review[3] finds scope 'for some major restructuring of IVB focusing on changes affecting entry to IVB, the value of the benefit in payment and the duration of receipt'. In other words: making it harder to claim, reducing the amount paid, and cutting the time claimants can receive it. One option is for 'more rigorous medical controls over access'. The path to a stricter assessment process is being laid.

On 4 June, a memo[4] describes a discussion between three senior civil servants on a 'scheme for the future control of invalidity benefit'. One of the trio is Dr Mansel Aylward.

Aylward had been a GP in Wales before founding a research company and being headhunted by the Department of Health and Social Security (DHSS) in 1985. He had been promoted in 1988 to deputy chief medical adviser. Aylward will be described as the architect of the new assessment process. It is, he tells me in 2023, his 'claim to fame'.

Aylward and his colleagues believe GPs should be sidelined. Instead, claimants should express their own views through self-assessment questions. They would then be examined by a doctor from the Benefits Agency Medical Service (BAMS), usually at an examination centre. A report, with a recommendation from the BAMS doctor, would be sent for a decision by a Benefits Agency adjudication officer, although the BAMS doctor might occasionally need 'to obtain further information either from the GP or sometimes from a consultant, or even from elsewhere'.

This request for further information would become known as seeking 'further medical evidence', and it would become a crucial and controversial stage of the claim process. The department's frequent refusal to ensure the necessary information is obtained from the healthcare professionals who know a benefit claimant best will, in future years, lead to the deaths of countless disabled people.

The 4 June memo provides a remarkably durable skeleton for how disabled people will be assessed for disability benefits over the next three decades.

Another memo the same month[5] highlights the arrogance of DSS's medical specialists. A Dr T. P. Scott tells Aylward that 'with IVB we are still in the Dark Ages'. He suggests a harsher approach, allowing someone to be found 'partially capable of work' and therefore eligible only for a lower rate of benefit. He claims 'too much power rests with people who don't know what they are doing'.

Scott says it is important to 'remove the GP from the equation', restricting them to 'confirming the diagnosis at the start of the claim … From then on it is up to us to give the medical opinion on capacity for work.' If this happens, tribunals would be likely to 'put less weight on any letter of support sent by a GP and, properly, pay more attention to the opinion of the experts, ie us!'.

Scott suggests selling this to the British Medical Association as a 'positive step forward'. 'The more conscientious amongst their number may even breathe a sigh of relief at the thought of not having to have further arguments with "malingerers" over yet another request for a certificate.' The consequences of this arrogance will be far-reaching.

Plans for a major review of IVB appear to have been swilling around the DSS corridors for at least a couple of years. Lilley – by now Lord Lilley – will tell me in 2022 that his recollection of the review's origin is 'somewhat vague'. But he agrees officials had probably 'been working on options to reform IB before I arrived'.

> I made it clear that I wanted to curb growth of spending on benefits without cutting the real level of benefits (I was under pressure from the Star Chamber to allow only a 2 per cent increase in line with public sector pay). So I decided to focus on those benefits which were increasing most rapidly. IB had trebled in a decade. But I was a bit suspicious of officials when they seemed almost eager to do something about it – suspecting that my very experienced predecessor, Tony Newton [who died in 2012] must have turned their plans down and they were to palm them off on me as a novice!

He adopts the key proposal, to introduce 'an objective medical test'. The review will examine restricting eligibility, limiting its duration, tightening 'medical control of claims', and achieving 'relatively significant savings'.

Lilley's department is set on a slow journey that will lead to tragedy. As Dr China Mills will point out, the harm caused to disabled claimants would not be seen in a moment of spectacular violence. It would build slowly, hidden from view. As Rob Nixon has written of environmental harm: 'By slow violence I mean a violence that occurs gradually and out of sight, a violence of delayed destruction that is dispersed across time and space, an attritional violence that is typically not viewed as violence at all.'

3

'Ignorant' Ministers, the Insurance Industry, and Lilley's Little List

On 22 July 1992, Alan Woods, private secretary to Peter Lilley, sends a memo[1] to a DSS colleague that will have a hugely significant impact on the disability benefits system.

> A note to confirm our telephone conversation.
>
> Secretary of State would like to know more about the approach of insurance companies to sickness insurance. He is keen that we should take on board any lessons which their practices may offer in our examination of how IVB expenditure can be restrained. Particular areas on which he would like to know more are:
>
> How do they assess claims to determine who qualifies for payments?
>
> What is their approach to medical examinations? Do they rely on GP's, who may have no incentive to curtail the length of the claim, or do they have alternatives?
>
> … As discussed, it may be best to sound out one or two insurers as part of the discussions A4 [a DSS department] will be having with them …

Mansel Aylward gathers material from various insurance companies. He claims later that he concluded there was nothing DSS could learn from them, and, if anything, 'they could learn from us'.

Whether or not DSS did learn some of their tricks and tactics – and later developments suggest they did – it is the beginning of a relationship that will see the insurance industry, and other parts of the private sector, develop an increasingly tight grip on both the policy and practice of disability assessments.

August 1992. A DSS memo[2] reports on an IVB 'brainstorming session' led by Aylward. There are 45 proposals, most of which are agreed. One suggestion is that GPs who allow too many incapacity claims should be 'identified', and even sanctioned. Another proposal sets the tone for future changes. For those who fail to attend an examination with 'no good cause', payment of benefit should stop 'immediately'. They should be asked to attend another examination 'only if the excuse is genuine'. Aylward will later insist he vetoed the suggestion, but the idea will eventually sit right at the heart of the department's hostile environment for claimants.

Now aged 80 and recently returned from an international lecture tour, Aylward will tell me he led the IVB reforms, and formed a group of about 40 advisers (DSS records suggest there were about 80 members), including disabled people. The aim, he says, was to 'define what it is that prevents people from working due to disability or impairment. I defined it. And yes, I did lead on it, because I felt we had to be giving the money to those that deserve [it] because they were incapable of work because of a disease, a mental illness or disability.'

I ask him whether these reforms originated with ministers, or civil servants like himself. When he arrived in London in 1988 he found ministers 'quite ignorant of the issues'. But he insists there was no pressure placed on any minister, although he detected no resistance. It was civil servants who came up with the ideas, but the reforms were 'driven by ministers'.

In October 1992, Peter Lilley writes to Michael Portillo.[3] 'Two key reasons for the growth in IVB expenditure have been an increase in the length of time people have stayed on the benefit and … its comparative generosity,' he tells him. He suggests it is right to 'tackle this difficult issue' with 'the reining back of expenditure long term as the big prize'.

Days later, Lilley delivers a set-piece speech at the Tory conference,[4] in which he pitches a crackdown on the 'something for nothing society'. He talks about fraudulent benefit claims, which are 'an insult to the law-abiding majority'. He speaks about 'bogus claims', 'spongers', 'locusts', and welfare being 'a way of life'. Lilley, in his pinstriped suit, flanked by rows of senior party figures, tells the conference: 'We are not in the business of subsidising scroungers.'

He sets out his plans for a welfare crackdown to 'I've Got a Little List', from Gilbert and Sullivan's *The Mikado*, a song performed in the comic opera by the Lord High Executioner. Benefit offenders, bogus claimants, and sponging socialists, 'they'd none of them be missed,' he tells a mostly delighted audience of Tory members, although some appear from their folded arms and grimaces to be appalled by his parody.

Aylward tells me in 2023 that Lilley 'never spoke to me in those terms' and never appeared obsessed with benefit fraud. He says he told Lilley he didn't agree with his conference speech, but he adds: 'Peter Lilley never struck me as a hard man. Whenever I said to him, "I think we shouldn't do that, or perhaps that's not fair," he agreed.'

Lilley tells me years later that he was not the first to 'identify the need to distinguish between those needing disability benefits and those needing help into work'. He claims many disabled people supported his efforts to recognise 'that some people abuse the system' and focus benefits on those who deserved them. He insists it was officials who convinced him 'the benefit was being awarded to claimants who were not really entitled to it … Officials convinced me that this was a genuine problem not vice versa.'

He denies he was 'scapegoating' claimants, a claim he describes as 'nonsense'. 'No-one suggests, or ever suggested, that most – let alone all – claimants are not really entitled to the benefit,' he says, although this hadn't been my suggestion. 'My reforms were designed to ensure that the benefit was focussed on those genuinely entitled to it by introducing an objective medical test.'

He says he had been 'very keen to avoid legal action' and so ensured DSS only classified 'a very small proportion of claims' as fraudulent. He claims this explains why he could not produce evidence of substantial levels of benefit fraud.

But Aylward disagrees. Fraud 'was a minor thing,' he tells me. 'The recent figures are, you know, probably around 3 per cent [of spending] or whatever. I agree with that, and my point is I wasn't concerned with fraud because fraud was a small item, and I didn't want to expend all my energy on a minor, minor issue.'

The following month, DSS civil servants send Lilley papers in preparation for a Commons speech.[5] They tell him to say that spending needs to be restricted 'to better reflect what the country can afford'. They claim spending on IVB is forecast to rise from under £2 billion in 1983–84 to more than £7 billion by 1994–95 if left 'unchecked', while recipients 'have risen from 760,000 in 1983–84 to 1,325,000 in 1991–92', and 'are forecast to go on rising'. There is 'no evidence that the nation's health has declined to this extent', and they must continue the policy of 'targeting available public money on disabled people in most need', a phrase that will crop up repeatedly in the decades ahead.

But there is no mention of other significant factors explaining the increases: life expectancy increasing for some conditions, more married women becoming entitled to receive IVB, and disabled people finding it harder to secure jobs. Mansel Aylward will tell me he agrees that many factors explained the rise in IVB spending.

DSS civil servants must have known their briefing was misleading, if only because of the earlier work of the National Audit Office which highlighted these other factors.

Lilley follows his officials' advice.[6] He tells MPs he has subjected the department's costs 'to rigorous examination' and is determined to 'tackle fraud and abuse of benefits'. He plans 'better targeted' tests, and 'more effective action' when people fail to attend their examination or are found fit for work. He has, he says, 'sought to curb programmes which might otherwise pre-empt the resources needed to sustain recovery in the longer term', which will 'protect benefits for those hit by the chill wind of world recession' and 'channel increased support to the most needy'. This scapegoating of disabled people – an accusation Lilley strongly denies – will be used repeatedly by future ministers and governments.

By April 1993, civil servants are finalising a submission for ministers.[7] They say incapacity benefits should 'look different and cost substantially less'. The assessment will be based 'solely on the medical condition', and they warn of 'a considerable amount of opposition since the clear effect would be to limit entitlement' through a 'considerable tightening of the qualifying conditions'.

The aim of the test 'will be to assess a claimant's capabilities against a range of activities involved in working', such as lifting, bending, and climbing. It is expected to exclude about 20 per cent of those who would qualify for IVB.

And there is another striking admission: 'We should aim to create an environment which encourages greater private sector provision.'

> LEAKED Whitehall documents last night revealed government plans both to tax invalidity benefit and to withhold it from up to 60,000 people.
>
> The proposals are in a draft letter to the Prime Minister from Peter Lilley, Secretary of State for Social Security.
>
> Benefit cuts, aimed at saving the Treasury £1.3 billion over the next seven years, were agreed at a meeting on Wednesday between Mr Lilley and Michael Portillo, Chief Secretary to the Treasury.
>
> In the letter that was faxed by mistake to the Press Association news agency, Mr Lilley says: 'I propose a three-pronged course of action which would focus the benefit more closely on the long-term sick, make it less generous and make it taxable.'
>
> He acknowledges the changes are 'bound to be controversial' and will cause 'some outrage'. (*The Independent*, 10 June 1993)

When John Major addresses this leak in prime minister's questions,[8] he says the government is 'entirely right' to consider IVB for cuts.

> The number of people receiving invalidity benefit has more than doubled during the past ten years from 700,000 to more than 1.5 million. Frankly, it beggars belief that so many more people have suddenly become invalids, especially at a time when the health of the population has improved. I make no apologies for looking at this area of expenditure.

Major ignores the many other explanations for the increase in IVB numbers.

But while civil servants and ministers are claiming the IVB system is too lenient and generous, disabled people are saying the opposite. A report shows continuing government attacks on IVB are creating a 'climate of fear' among disabled people.[9] Disability charities Disability Alliance and RADAR surveyed more than 300 claimants, with 80 per cent saying GPs sometimes or often refuse sick notes to people who advisers consider unfit for work. Medical examinations, which only last ten minutes on average, are often 'stressful and painful', with doctors frequently missing key details.

In July, Peter Lilley delivers the annual Mais Lecture,[10] a significant event for the City of London. He says growth in social security spending is beginning to 'outstrip the nation's ability to pay'. He warns of 'benefit dependency', and the need to 'safeguard' the 'most vulnerable'. But he also speaks about the role the private sector – the pension and insurance industries – should play, and the importance of people making 'private provision for their own security'. It is another sign of the insurance industry's growing hold over the department.

4

Scapegoats, the All Work Test, and How Ill-health Became a Luxury

While disabled people are already warning of the IVB 'climate of fear', the department knows the best way to secure public backing for its cuts and reforms is to scapegoat those who rely on that support.

It is January 1994, and the government is publishing its new Social Security (Incapacity for Work) Bill. Peter Lilley tells MPs[1] that invalidity benefit will be replaced by incapacity benefit and 'a new and more objective test of incapacity for work', which will focus on those 'genuinely too unwell to work' and ensure the benefit is 'affordable'. He insists this is 'not an attack on the sick and disabled' but 'designed to protect their benefit against those who abuse it ... People who work for a modest wage resent seeing neighbours, apparently as fit as themselves, living on invalidity benefit.' He says his new test will be simpler to understand and easier to apply, and that the approach is 'highly respected by disabled people and their representatives'. But DSS will soon be receiving responses from disability organisations to a consultation on the new test, and they will not be supportive.

Aylward's new 'all work test' will usually be applied after 28 weeks of sickness or disability, with the claimant sent a questionnaire to assess their 'long-term incapacity for work'. Their GP will be asked for a 'diagnosis of their illness and the principal disabling conditions' but not about their ability to work. Most cases will be looked at by BAMS, with just over half of claimants expected to be called for an assessment. The number of examinations is expected to rise from 300,000 a year to 700,000, with another 680 doctors to be recruited.

One crucial difference is a new points-based system to decide eligibility. But Professor Nick Wikeley, later to be a social security upper tribunal judge,[2] says the new test will remain subjective and will focus only on 'medical incapacity', excluding factors such as age and experience. Many new claimants will receive 'considerably less', and more will be found fit for work. Government policy, says Wikeley, 'is clearly to encourage private provision for the risks traditionally safeguarded by social security'. That is: insurance. The government's new benefit, he says, reaffirms the division between the 'deserving' and the 'undeserving' poor.

As disabled academic Jenny Morris will point out years later,[3] none of this is new. 'Those administering the Poor Law in the seventeenth century were concerned to weed out "sturdy vagabonds" from making claims on public resources, and distinctions have been made between the "deserving" and "undeserving" ever since.'

DSS issues a consultation on the new all work test. The responses[4] begin to highlight multiple concerns, including many that will be repeatedly raised and ignored over the next three decades.

Disability Alliance raises concerns about 'the impact of a purely "functional" approach on people with fluctuating conditions, less visible disabilities, and mental health problems', and concludes: 'Not only is the proposed test wrong in principle, it will have unfair and arbitrary results in practice.'

The Royal Association for Disability and Rehabilitation (RADAR) refutes the claim that the increase in IVB numbers is due to 'inappropriate claims and "lead swingers"'. It points to its research with Disability Alliance which found no evidence of 'malingering'.

The Law Society warns BAMS doctors will be put in a position 'where they may risk failing to meet proper professional standards by being asked to make decisions without access to adequate information, in particular medical records or other relevant medical data', particularly when assessing people with learning difficulties, mental distress, or chronic pain.

The Convention of Scottish Local Authorities asks DSS how a 'snap-shot' assessment can truly determine if a claimant is 'fit for work'. It warns of 'arbitrary results for many claimants', particularly – again – those with learning difficulties or mental distress.

Others say the test ignores stress, pain, and fatigue, that BAMS doctors will not be suitably trained, that DSS is wrong to reduce the role of GPs, and that the process discriminates against those who are not good at speaking up for themselves.

The department makes some adjustments in response, deciding that claimants with a 'severe mental health condition' will not have to complete a questionnaire or be examined, while no claimant undergoing treatment for mental distress will be found fit for work 'without further information first being sought from their GP or psychiatrist'. The bill passes through parliament.

Looking ahead 30 years, the same concerns are still being raised, with the same stubborn refusal of civil servants and politicians to listen. But even those raising concerns in the early months of 1994 are not warning that the assessment will cause countless deaths. That will come later.

The assessment had been due to be launched at a press conference. But Treasury officials have 'expressed some concerns about the possible reactions to the proposals'.[5] Instead, there is a press release.[6] The test will be based on a person's ability to perform a series of work-related activities and 'will involve defined areas of function of the body and mind'. Each function will have ranked levels of severity – known as descriptors. At or above those levels it would be 'unreasonable to expect the person to work'.

William Hague, minister for social security, says the assessment is 'vital if we are to ensure that benefit is targeted on people who are genuinely sick and disabled and unable to work', and – if that wasn't clear enough – will 'focus help on those for whom it was always intended, people who are genuinely sick and disabled'.

Meanwhile, *The Guardian* warns the reforms mean 'ill-health will become a luxury', that disabled people 'face a poorer, bleaker future' and – helpfully for the insurance industry – many employees 'are likely to turn increasingly to private permanent health insurance to guard their future income'.[7]

The government's primary message is clear: the test will weed out frauds and scroungers. The secondary message is also clear: if you can afford it, take out private insurance.

Weeks later, Peter Lilley receives a memo[8] from John Arbury, a senior DSS civil servant. He says a 'significant number remain concerned', with some 'not convinced that the test will be a fair assessment of incapacity'. But DSS civil servants are nothing if not stubborn and complacent, and Arbury adds: 'Each issue raised has been considered previously – nothing new was raised.'

5

Periodic Purges, Unum, and Selective Use of Evidence

6 April 1995. John Major is in his place halfway along the mahogany cabinet table. Major sits at its widest point, like all prime ministers, so he can see all his ministers, a necessary precaution given the political manoeuvrings blighting his term in office. To Major's right are Peter Lilley and fellow Thatcherite Michael Portillo, the employment secretary. Others present include chancellor Kenneth Clarke, Michael Heseltine, president of the Board of Trade, and home secretary Michael Howard.

Lilley tells his colleagues[1] that, from 13 April, sickness benefit and invalidity benefit will be replaced by the new incapacity benefit. He says the changes are necessary because the number of people receiving IVB has doubled over the last ten years. The existing benefits are poorly targeted and put GPs in the 'invidious' position of effectively determining the rate at which their patients receive benefit.

The most significant change, Lilley says, will be the introduction of a new medical test, which will focus incapacity benefit on people who are 'genuinely' incapable of working. He says it is likely that about 20 per cent of those who previously qualified for invalidity benefit will not do so under incapacity benefit, and that within two years about 240,000 people who had formerly received invalidity benefit will be found capable of work. Lilley says his reforms are likely to attract controversy when apparently deserving cases have their benefits cut.

The cabinet discuss Lilley's presentation. There are concerns about adverse publicity, and the possibility that GPs will talk to journalists about patients wrongly found fit to work. But no minister raises concerns about the risk of harm to those disabled people who will be put through the new assessment process and found unfairly fit for work.

One of the things Lilley doesn't tell his fellow ministers is that his department has been discussing 'possible contingency action' in case the new test is 'ineffective, unworkable or unpopular'.[2] The back-up plan is to return to the existing IVB assessment, which would have 'major political, financial and operational implications'.

Meanwhile, a columnist in *Disability Now* magazine[3] says invalidity benefit has not been as lax as politicians suggest. Dave Gibbs describes 'periodic purges' aimed at forcing people off the benefit. 'Two years ago, this was cranked up to a new pitch, and thousands of people had their benefit stopped,' he says. 'The tightening up was so indiscriminate that, in one county alone, there were 800 appeals against loss of benefit and over 90 per cent of them were successful. Clearly, enough savings could not be made within the present rules, so in April the rules change.'

Lilley's scrounger rhetoric is never far from the surface. In May, he tells MPs[4] they should not be intimidated by disabled people protesting about incapacity benefit. 'People on our television screens who have been refused benefit,' he says, 'will be seen for the first time in their lives in a wheelchair.'

In June, renowned investigative journalist Paul Foot publishes an article in *Private Eye*[5] that appears to have been the first to expose the key role the insurance industry is playing in incapacity benefit reform. Foot reveals that Lilley has hired Dr John LoCascio from US corporation Unum Life Insurance to advise on his reforms. This is three years after Lilley first told his officials he wanted 'to know more about the approach of insurance companies to sickness insurance'. Unum had bought the Dorking-based National Employers' Life Assurance Company (NEL) in 1990, changing its name to Unum Ltd, providing a major foothold in the UK market.

Aylward will later tell me that LoCascio looked like the actor Danny DeVito and 'was a chap who was intellectually excellent and had great experience in looking at disability and assessment'. Although he didn't recommend him to Lilley, he approved the appointment. 'I thought he was an asset. You know, we bounced things off him,' he tells me in 2023.

Unum's chairman, Ward E. Graffam, had admitted Unum would gain from the reforms in the company's 1994 annual report: 'The impending changes to the State ill-health benefits system heralded in the November 1993 Budget will create unique sales opportunities across the entire disability market and we will be launching a concerted effort to harness the potential in these.'

Foot says Unum took advantage of the reforms with an advertising campaign timed to coincide with the introduction of incapacity benefit in April 1995. One ad stated: 'April 13, unlucky for some. Because tomorrow the new rules on state incapacity benefit announced in the 1993 autumn budget come into effect. Which means that if you fall ill and have to rely on state incapacity benefit, you could be in serious trouble.'

LoCascio was a member of Lilley's 'medical evaluation group', whose task was to 'monitor and validate the quality standards for the doctors involved in the all-work assessments'. He was also paid £40,000 a year to help train doctors in the new assessment techniques. It is difficult to square this with Aylward's insistence that DSS learned nothing from the insurance industry.

The Treasury is pressing DSS to make greater savings. It picks up on the earliest reported results from the all work test. By 31 May, only 28 people have 'failed' the test and been found fit for work. A Treasury official says this 'does not seem like very many'. DSS officials accept[6] – without admitting this to the Treasury – that the initial results are 'clearly disappointing'. The Treasury had also asked about the apparent absence of 'critical reports in the press' and whether DSS 'noticed any signs of the trouble Mr Lilley has been expecting'.[7] In the DSS response, an official warns that 'hard cases reaching the press may emerge at any time within the coming months'.

The following month, a paper[8] written by LoCascio and Aylward, by now DSS's chief medical adviser, argues that those sick and disabled people who wish to claim out-of-work disability benefits or from disability insurance policies 'may require specialist investigation, treatment, and documentation' that is not available to most doctors. The paper shows again how DSS, its incapacity benefit reforms, and the insurance industry are closely intertwined.

Aylward and LoCascio stress the importance of disability assessment medicine, a new specialism they will do much to promote, and the profession of disability analysts who can be trained to assess 'fitness for work'. They insist it is possible to identify and address 'subjective questions' around a person's 'functional capacities'. They try to build a case for their version of the biopsychosocial (BPS) model of disability, which many will argue puts the blame for disability on the disabled person, rather than the barriers they face in society or the impairment or health condition itself.

LoCascio and Aylward argue that a 'comprehensive psychiatric evaluation' of the claimant is vital because the person's own subjective attitude towards their illness can lead them to exaggerate their restrictions. The role of doctors, they say, is to describe the claimant's health condition. The analyst's job is to work out if the claimant is 'genuinely' unable to work.

Aylward will tell me, in 2023, that he had been 'plagued' by people arguing that his BPS model blamed disabled people for their disability, which he says is 'rubbish'.

> I've got people painting on my house on the doors. I've had people letting tyres down on my car. I've had people writing abusive letters to me. All of which are completely unfounded. I really get very, very upset by these people who are doing this damage to me. They've published in America and on the continent in French saying I'm a charlatan. That's not fair.

The BPS approach will become interwoven with the government's rhetoric. Sometimes it will be subtle, sometimes not so subtle. But the inference will remain: that many claimants of incapacity benefits are malingering.

* * *

It was, the National Audit Office (NAO) will say six years later,[9] the 'inadequacies' of the assessments provided by the Benefits Agency

Medical Services (BAMS) that persuaded ministers to outsource the assessment process to the private sector.

This was a time when the private sector was taking advantage of the Conservative government's enthusiasm for outsourcing.[10] In December 1995, ministers announce their decision to outsource benefit assessments. They ask DSS officials to award a contract by April 1997. Initially, 33 companies express an interest, before this is reduced to a shortlist of five.[11]

As disabled activist and author Ellen Clifford will write years later,[12] outsourcing the assessment process will allow the government 'to cloud transparency and pass the buck', and it will let politicians 'conveniently blame providers' for wrongful assessment decisions. The decision is made just three years after Peter Lilley invited the insurance industry to prowl the corridors of the DSS.

In January 1996, Alistair Burt, who has taken over from William Hague as minister for disabled people, writes to Lilley.[13] He warns that the social security committee is suggesting there is a 'conceptual flaw' in the all work test. There are concerns about the number of successful appeals. He also says publication of an evaluation of the test will 'need care' as it suggests a significant proportion of doctors disagree over whether a claimant is fit for work. He suggests delaying the release of the findings.

By the end of the first year, ministers are concerned at the low number of claimants being found fit for work, and they want to 'accelerate the process so that disallowances occur as early as possible'.

They devise three projects to trial proposed changes, and a review of the reforms.[14]

Neil Couling – a senior DSS civil servant who will play a significant role in the universal credit reforms of the 2010s – says the review means the incapacity benefit reform process will 'retain a high profile' after an implementation that has so far 'gone very quietly'.

The DSS argument was that the growth in incapacity benefits was out of control, with the number of claimants rising since the early 1970s at a time when the nation's health was improving. But researcher and consultant Steve Griffiths will write later that the case for reform was 'based from the beginning on selective use of evidence'.[15]

He analyses ONS trends on people with limiting long-term illness. It shows the number in the 16–44 age group rose by half from 1975 to 1995–96, and those aged 45–64 increased by nearly a quarter. 'This is surely one important factor in explaining the increase in claims for incapacity benefit,' he says.

He suggests that improvements in medical science and its application across the NHS led to more people needing and being eligible for incapacity benefits. Griffiths will also point to a decrease in these numbers between 1995–96 and 2008 (a fall of a fifth for those 16–44, and a fall of 13 per cent for those 45–64), a time when the number of those claiming the new incapacity benefit was falling. The figures suggest that the introduction of incapacity benefit may have been based on a fatal misunderstanding, or even a reckless disregard, of developments in the nation's health.

* * *

DSS ministers are sent a briefing pack in March 1996 as they approach incapacity benefit's first anniversary.[16] It includes a startling fact: of the 27,719 former recipients of incapacity benefit who are now claiming unemployment benefits after being reassessed as fit for work, only 289 have started jobs. This figure is marked 'use only if required'. Ministers will not want to explain why so many disabled people found fit for work are finding it so difficult to secure jobs.

There are other concerning figures in the briefing pack. In the first year of incapacity benefit, the number of claimants is expected to fall by 30,000 to 1,830,000, while spending is projected to drop from £7.8 billion in 1995–96 to £7.2 billion in 1996–97 and £6.7 billion in 1997–98.

Ministers are briefed on how to respond if asked about claimants with mental distress, the appointment of Unum's John LoCascio, the contracting out of assessments, or private insurance. 'Individuals should be able to choose whether to make additional provision,' they are told to say, and: 'Permanent Health Insurance can play an important part in some people's long-term planning.' The interests of the insurance industry are now embedded within DSS.

DSS invites expressions of interest in the incapacity benefit assessment contract, which will be split into three regions. But incapacity benefit reform has not taken place in a vacuum. Legislation is passed to reform unemployment benefits, with the new jobseeker's allowance introduced in October. As Tom O'Grady says,[17] the need for claimants to 'actively' look for work has been 'given teeth', with more 'intensive' checks by DSS staff. Claimants also need to sign a formal contract laying out their responsibilities, and there are compulsory fortnightly interviews, with tough sanctions for those not doing enough.

'It marked the true beginning of welfare-to-work in the UK,' says O'Grady, 'and the re-emergence of the strong conditionality of the 1920s–30s.'

It will also have a profound impact on disabled people, both those forced onto jobseeker's allowance after being found fit for work, but also those in the future who will face strict conditions for receiving out-of-work disability benefits. The consequences will emerge slowly, but the impact will be deadly.

* * *

While Lilley and his civil servants have been introducing incapacity benefit, a BBC documentary team has been invited inside the blue-carpeted corridors of the department's Richmond House headquarters, and the nearby Adelphi, with its Art Deco marble entrance lobby and grand staircases, where Aylward and his Benefits Agency team are based.

Filming begins in 1995 and the first episode of the five-part series airs in September 1996.[18] There is access to Peter Lilley, who fidgets in front of the cameras, and the grey-haired Aylward, who is much more assured about his new, 'more objective' assessment.

Much of the series is government propaganda, stressing the rising cost of the social security safety net and hinting at widespread fraud. Invalidity benefit 'is known to cynics as the bad back benefit', viewers are told. It points out that someone found fit for work faces a fall in benefits from £73 to £45.70 a week.

In the final episode – dedicated to incapacity benefit – one doctor who will be assessing claimants says he suspects 'a lot of people perhaps are swinging the lead just a wee bit'. But another doctor, also filmed at DSS's Glasgow medical centre, challenges the BBC's line of questioning. 'When you get the odd malingerer are you good at spotting them?' he is asked. He replies: 'I think malingerer's the wrong term. I don't think any of these people are malingering … it's an inflammatory term.' He adds later: 'Instead of sitting here trying to get people off benefits, we should really be out trying to improve people's housing and improve people's education and trying to improve industry.'

Meanwhile, *Disability Now* magazine reports[19] a disabled woman left with broken bones after undergoing the all work test. The woman, who has spondylosis affecting her spine and neck, was asked to kneel down, but could not get back to her feet. The Benefits Agency doctor refused to help, and as she was trying to get up, she broke bones in her hand. The doctor turned her back and walked away. But worse is to come.

6

The Death of David Holmes, and the Causal Link

'All the evidence is that it is working as intended,' ministers had been briefed in March 1996, as they prepared to mark the first anniversary of incapacity benefit. 'No evidence of problems with the test.' But there were problems, particularly for 54-year-old David Holmes.

In March 1982, David had a massive heart attack. The former Royal Marine had worked as a hydraulic fitter at British Steel in Ebbw Vale, Gwent, and at a furniture factory in nearby Cwmtillery. He had lived most of his life in Cwmtillery. He was a popular member of Abertillery Orpheus Male Choir, and a keen Citizens Band radio operator, with his equipment kept in a shed at the bottom of his garden. From his garden, he can look across the valley at the young fir trees growing on the hillside previously scarred by Cwmtillery Colliery, which closed in 1982. At the end of the street stand two former pit head wheels, encased in the same stone used to build the former National Coal Board cottages.

By 1996, David – Dai, as his friends know him – has been divorced for more than 25 years. He enjoys fishing with friends, but the most exercise he can manage is a short walk in Cwmtillery Lakes, just across the road, with his beloved cocker spaniel.

After his heart attack, David was granted a lifetime mobility pension. But on 14 October, thanks to Peter Lilley's incapacity benefit reforms, he is told to appear before a DSS doctor in nearby Pontllanfraith for a medical examination.

The assessment takes less than 40 minutes. He needs 15 points to qualify for incapacity benefit. But the doctor grants him just seven points for being unable to walk more than 200 metres 'without stopping or severe discomfort'. For the other eleven 'physical disabilities' functions – including lifting and carrying, bending and kneeling, and getting up from a chair – he is granted zero points. Less than two weeks later, on 26 October, he is told to return his mobility pension book to the DSS. He withdraws his final payment two days later. On 4 November, he writes to the Benefits Agency:

Dear Sir/Madam
I wish to appeal against the adjudication assessment concerning my ability to resume work, on the grounds that with the state of my health I know that I am medically unfit to resume working.

Secondly I am convinced that this assessment is based not on the state of my health but is purely and simply a political issue. We are all aware of the forthcoming General Election, indeed, it is all we seem to read about in the media and see on television. We are also aware of the Government statement saying 'We will get the long term unemployed back to work'... they did not add 'At any cost'.

Prior to March 1982, I had a reputation as a good workman, and was also actively involved in sport, running my own judo club for 12 years for the benefit of local youngsters, which incidentally I did voluntarily without payment. On recovering in hospital after suffering a massive coronary, I was told by Dr Rajah that if I had not been as fit as I was, then I would never have survived the heart attack. When I was finally discharged from the hospital, after many weeks of examinations and tests, I asked Mr Thomas, the consultant, at Nevill Hall Hospital, what the long term effects of the coronary might be and how soon I could resume work. He said, and I quote: 'You can forget about work, as you will never work again, the reason being, if you have another coronary like the last one, you will never survive it.' Unquote.

Over the next few years I was sent to see three independent doctors ... These doctors agreed on one salient point – I was medically unfit for work. I was then granted a Mobility Pension for the rest of my life.

Which brings me to the one and only point on which I and the adjudicator seem to agree: I have a mobility problem. Form 1B-65A states 'Cannot walk more than 200m without stopping or severe dis-

comfort.' (On a bad day I cannot leave the house.) This is the precise reason why I was granted the Mobility Pension!

My mobility problems are caused by respiratory problems, which are caused by angina, which, in turn, is a direct result of the coronary thrombosis!!!

How can a doctor, who I saw for less than 40 minutes, and who asked the most irrelevant questions – 'What TV programmes do you watch?' and 'What books do you read?' – and a DSS adjudication officer, make an assessment on the state of my health and state that I am medically able to return to work, based on a questionnaire, which was hardly relevant to my particular circumstances?

They have never seen me on a bad day on the edge of my bed, trying to get my breath before I can even dress, trying to control my breathing before I can make a cup of tea ... Contrary to that stated on form IB-65A, LIFTING AND CARRYING, my friend and his wife do all my weekly shopping for me as I am unable to carry heavy shopping bags without getting chest pains ...

I would like nothing better than to have my health restored, have a job of work, with a decent living wage and live a normal life like other people. Instead, I get very frustrated and depressed. I fail to see why I should have to risk another coronary and therefore risk my life to further the political aspirations of Government bureaucrats.

Yours faithfully,

David Holmes

Dai's closest friends are Pauline and Dennis Johnson, the couple he refers to in his letter. They have a cocker spaniel from the same litter and walk them together by Cwmtillery Lakes. Dai met Pauline when she was out with a 'gang of girls' from work. They soon realised Dai was in the choir with her husband. The three of them became close, and Pauline would drive Dai's mother, Dolly, to church on a Sunday evening. Pauline would help Dai look after his mother and help him with his own housework.

'You couldn't meet a better fella than Dai Holmes,' Pauline, now aged 82, would tell me years later. 'If he could do you a good turn, he would do it, no matter what he had to go through. If he had to risk his own life, he would do it. I cried on his shoulder many a time.'

After his benefits are stopped, Dai will often talk to the Johnsons about being found fit for work. 'It was so unfair,' says Pauline. 'He wasn't able to go to work. No way.' He was constantly worrying about how he would pay his bills. 'He was worried sick, how he was going to pay this, and how was he going to pay that. He didn't know what to do.'

Every week, Dai attends a meeting with the Johnsons of their local Citizens Band radio club. The day after writing the letter to the Benefits Agency, Dai attends a Bonfire Night party hosted by one of the group's members. Pauline drives him there. But halfway through the party, he tells her he doesn't feel well and asks her to drive him home.

They have just passed the Aberbeeg ambulance station when Dai slumps forward with his hands across his chest. Pauline makes a U-turn and speeds back to the ambulance station. She tells the *Gwent Gazette* later: 'He wasn't moving or breathing so the ambulance men put him in the back of an ambulance and tried to revive him. After about 20 minutes they took him to Nevill Hall but nothing could be done.'

'They took him in the ambulance and when we got to the hospital ... they told me he had passed away and he'd gone,' she remembers now. 'That was it, he'd gone.' The letter to the DSS is still waiting to be posted at Dai's home in Cwmtillery.

The Johnsons find the letter and show it to the *Gwent Gazette*.[1] 'David had been worried sick about going to the medical,' Pauline tells the paper. 'After finding out he had lost his benefit David was a changed man ... He said the DSS hadn't listened to anything he had told them.' The *Gazette*'s front-page coverage is headlined 'Worried to Death'.

Hundreds attend his funeral at Abertillery Tabernacle Chapel. Pauline and Den sort out Dai's affairs, and arrange for his estate to be passed to his daughter, who lives a few miles away with his ex-wife. Pauline and Den buy a bench overlooking Cwmtillery Lakes in Dai's memory.

Pauline was devastated by Dai's death. She found it particularly difficult when she was in her car. 'Every time I got in that car, I used to see him sat in the front seat.' Eventually she gave it to her son.

Pauline has no doubt the stress of the 'fit for work' decision caused his death. 'He would be here now today if that hadn't happened,' she tells me.

The *Gazette*'s coverage has alerted the local Labour MP Llew Smith, who knew David and writes to DSS, enclosing a copy of the front-page story. Smith describes the 'sadness and anger' felt at David's death, and he delivers a fierce attack on the new assessment. One disabled constituent had been forced to 'grovel on the floor at the feet of the examiner' to see if she could pick up a piece of paper, even though she said it would cause her 'extreme pain'. Another constituent recovering from life-threatening surgery had been left with 'a severe disability' and was 'flabbergasted' to have his mobility benefits withdrawn. 'Health problems such as these are not unusual in Blaenau Gwent,' he says. 'Deaths from lung cancer, respiratory and heart disease are all above the national and county average.' Instead of responding positively to these health problems, he says, the government is 'pressuring people like David Holmes' and 'stigmatising them by giving the impression they have been fiddling the system'.

Llew Smith secures a late-night adjournment debate.[2] Only two MPs speak in the debate on 3 December: Smith and Alistair Burt, the minister for disabled people.

Smith describes Lilley's all work test as 'a degrading experience, conducted in an uncaring manner and introduced by the government with no concern for the health and well-being of the individual'. David Holmes, he says, was a 'much-loved and respected member of the community', and his letter had been 'an expression of the stress he experienced and the hopelessness he felt at the failure of the DSS to appreciate the true extent of his illness'. The government's only aim in introducing the 'all work test' was to cut costs, he says.

Burt insists David Holmes was correctly found fit for work. 'The arrangements for dealing with claims for incapacity benefit have been carefully designed,' he says. 'They ensure that all relevant information is taken into account, and in particular that people with severe medical conditions are dealt with sensitively.'

> Can the honourable gentleman tell me of a medical technique to predict a death from heart disease within five days? If he can, perhaps we can incorporate it in the test ... While we all deeply regret the death of Mr Holmes, from the information that we have we do not believe that it can be attributed to the application of the all work test.

Smith dismisses the minister's excuses. He says he knows how to anticipate if someone will die if they return to work.

> Just speak to the people who were responsible for David – the medical team and the consultants who said that, if David returned to work, history would repeat itself. Indeed, they said that the situation would be even more severe, and David would die. Those consultants were found to be right. David was found to be right.

The argument will be made repeatedly by critics of successive governments' assessment processes over the next three decades. How can someone given such a short period of time to assess someone's fitness for work possibly over-rule the expert evidence of doctors and consultants with detailed knowledge of the claimant's health?

The Commons debate ends, but discussion of David Holmes's death continues within DSS. The day before the debate, Dr Moira Henderson, medical quality coordinator for BAMS, had told colleagues[3] that David Holmes received 'an appropriate assessment'. The doctor who examined him was 'very experienced, very considerate, totally objective' and one of the best assessors in Wales. Following the debate, Burt is briefed that David Holmes's 'functional capacity was not reduced to a level where he would be rendered incapable of doing any type of work'.

Burt writes to Llew Smith.[4] He insists there is 'no question of quotas being set for the number of people who will be found fit for work'. A 'thorough examination' has 'not shown that the BAMS doctor made any serious error of judgement', and any 'causal link' between the decision to find him fit for work and his death 'must remain entirely speculative'.

Alistair Burt is not as confident about the test's safety as he has suggested, and he writes to Aylward,[5] mentioning other cases in which claimants have been found fit for work despite 'the presence of serious heart disease'.

Aylward assures him[6] there is nothing to be concerned about and says he is 'satisfied that the training and guidance given to approved doctors takes sufficient account of the assessment of people with heart disease' and that there is no 'substantial evidence that approved doctors are not following the guidance'.

Burt will tell me years later that, from his father's experience as a GP in Bury, he knew 'medical incapacity in a northern industrial town was real, and that heart disease and respiratory issues were a feature of our way of life and working, and our atmosphere in the damp northwest'. He says he brought this experience to his ministerial work.

He says he wanted the test to work 'with maximum sensitivity and care, but I knew that some decisions would be very fine', and he adds: 'I also knew that what befell people after government or official decisions would inevitably be ascribed to such decisions, whatever the true cause might actually be.' Although he had 'particular concerns about the impact of the test on those with heart conditions', he claims he was 'in no position, once my enquiries were answered by senior officials, to query the position further, unless new evidence arose'.

Aylward tells me he did not remember the David Holmes case, but he said he knew the department 'always had trouble with people who had had heart attacks, because we knew that if you had a heart attack, it didn't follow that you would have another one because you'd received treatment'.

When I suggest this was another case of DSS assessors thinking they knew better than consultants and other medical experts, he tells me: 'They may do, actually.' He eventually accepts that if David Holmes was, on some days, too unwell to leave the house, he probably should have been found not fit for work. But he insists that 'just one isolated case' does not show the system was 'wrong'.

The all work test evaluation findings are finally published in February 1997. Ministers had decided the results would be 'given a low profile publication' – delayed for more than a year – because of the 'complexity of the findings and the potential for them to be misinterpreted'.[7] The evaluation found that in only three out of four cases (76 per cent) did two doctors agree on whether a claimant was fit for work. The overall scores varied even more often. In fact, the scores on 'physical' elements were identical in only 32 per cent of cases, while the mental health scores were identical in just 11 per cent. Overall, the incapacity benefit test appears to be 'both reliable and valid' in just two-thirds of cases.

Burt writes to Frank Field, the Labour MP and chair of the Commons social security committee.[8] He says changes to the test have been made, including to the training provided to the doctors carrying out the tests and to the assessment, and that the evaluation was carried out when the test had only been in operation for about six months. He suggests the 76 per cent finding was 'encouraging'. He reassures Field that the all work test 'is capable of producing reliable medical advice and is a valid means to assess incapacity for work for the benefit assessment purposes for which it was intended'. But there is soon further confirmation that Lilley's all work test is not fit for purpose.

The National Association of Citizens Advice Bureaux (NACAB) publishes a report in March 1997,[9] based on evidence from 227 branches across England, Wales, and Northern Ireland. It reveals that government figures show that, of the 60 per cent of claimants who appeal against being 'disallowed' incapacity benefit, more than half eventually have it reinstated after they appeal.

Bureaux evidence, says the report, 'suggests that many persons who are in poor health are being caused anxiety, distress and pain by the operation of the All Work Test'. Some of the evidence that emerges from individual CABs is striking.

A bureau in Yorkshire describes three cases 'where it appeared that the doctor had determined clients' ability to walk up and down stairs by the ease with which they got onto and off the examining couch'.

A bureau in Wales 'reported a client with arthritis of the spine who explained she could not raise her arms above her head. The examining officer promptly held her arms and physically raised them above her head, and despite her cry of pain, recorded "no significant limitation" under the "reaching" category.'

There were concerns, too, about the way disabled people with mental distress were examined. A bureau in the West Midlands reported the case of a client with depression. The BAMS doctor failed to ask about the depression – even though it was the only condition on her sick note – other than to ask what medication she was taking. She failed the test, which left her suicidal. 'She was constantly in tears and contemplating how to take her own life.'

Another bureau reported a client with a history of mental distress, including a period in hospital, who was not examined by the BAMS doctor but simply told he 'ought to be out earning some money'.

The problems, warns NACAB chief executive Ann Abraham, 'can only get worse when such monitoring as currently exists is allowed to go by the board, as it almost certainly will do when medical services are contracted out'.

DSS dismisses the report.[10] It raises no new issues, is 'largely based on anecdotal evidence from claimants visiting CAB offices', and the issues are 'sporadic' or 'isolated', while NACAB 'produced exactly the same sort of evidence' with invalidity benefit, ministers are told in a memo.

In the same month the NACAB report is published, and just three months after the adjournment debate on the death of David Holmes, two more cases will demonstrate the all work test's fatal flaws.

The first I find referred to in a memo written on 12 March.[11] It is sent to Lilley, Burt, and other ministers. It warns of an 'apparent suicide of customer after failing the "All Work Test"'. Robert Parry, the left-wing MP for Liverpool Riverside, has contacted his local DSS office to call for an investigation. The claimant's name is 39-year-old Kevin Shields. The details are brief. BAMS was 'unable to certify that the customer was suffering from a severe mental health problem'.

Shields 'failed' the all work test and lodged an appeal. He had been receiving income support since the previous September due to depression, but this was cut by 20 per cent after he was found fit to work. Before a tribunal could hear his appeal, he took his own life.

The department is conducting a 'full investigation', and a hand-written note from Burt says he wants 'to be kept informed every step of the way'. The letter from Parry is not included in papers released by the National Archives, and neither are the results of the investigation. There is no mention of the case in parliament, possibly because John Major calls a general election just five days after the memo was written. When I approach the Liverpool and Wirral coroner's office for details of the inquest, 26 years later, it declines to release any papers to me as I am 'not classed as a "Properly Interested Person" in this case'.

On 24 March, another memo is sent to ministers.[12] This time, when approached in 2023, the coroner for West Yorkshire releases papers from the inquest to me. Dermot Kevin Comiskey, also known as John Comiskey, a 56-year-old divorced labourer from Dewsbury, West Yorkshire, had been receiving income support because of a back complaint. His GP had advised BAMS there was also an 'underlying psychiatric condition associated with alcohol and/or substance abuse, and a previous attempted suicide in 1995'. But BAMS said Comiskey 'could not be certified as suffering from a severe mental illness' and issued him with a questionnaire so he could describe how his conditions affected him. He failed to return the form or respond to a reminder.

The memo says BAMS should have been asked whether his benefits should be removed, but wasn't. His support was 'disallowed' on 13 November 1996, just a week after the death of David Holmes, but he continued to receive income support until 14 January 1997. He had made a fresh claim on 14 November and the decision to allow payment was made on 20 January, but because of confusion over his address, this was not implemented. He had appeared 'very depressed' during his last visit to the jobcentre. He told a receptionist he had had a tough few weeks because his girlfriend had taken her own life over Christmas.

He remained without benefits from 15 January until he was found dead at his home on 5 February. Again, the department says it is 'investigating the circumstances of this case to determine whether there are any lessons to be learned'.

The coroner's records reveal that an inquest was held on 16 April 1997, and it concludes that he took his own life 'whilst concerned about his personal circumstances'. The papers confirm that his partner had taken her own life the previous September. A friend told the inquest that she had seen him on the Thursday before he died when he had been 'very quiet, very withdrawn' and told her and her husband that his 'invalidity … had been stopped'.

She told the inquest: '… then he just shocked both me and my husband by saying, "Have you any idea how I can go about getting some food?"' They had fed him, and she fed him again when he visited again the following Monday. Two days later, she knocked on the unlocked door of his flat and found him dead.

Commenting on a written statement given by a Benefits Agency customer service manager, the coroner said it was clear there were 'money problems', which appeared to have been 'capable of clarification if Mr Comiskey had responded to various notifications from the Department'.

So here are two suicides, both linked to the all work test, being investigated by DSS. Civil servants and ministers will surely be wondering if there are others.

Alistair Burt tells me he remembers the two deaths. 'Claims or suggestions that a benefit decision was responsible for a suicide affects everyone involved in the chain of decision making, personally and painfully, as it did me and those working with me.' He says he would have added his hand-written note to the memo 'because of my interest and concern, not only about his situation but of others. I would be looking for anything new to enable changes to be made.'

The archive records I unearthed failed to reveal the results of any investigations carried out by the department, or whether information about these fatal flaws was passed by civil servants to the next government. But DSS and ministers will surely be aware that this is not the first time suicides have been linked to a national programme to cut spending on disability benefits.

In the early 1980s, Ronald Reagan instigated a regime of cuts to disabled people's out-of-work benefits.[13] In 1982 and 1983, the *New York Times* later reported[14] on a series of suicides of disabled people who had been told they were losing these benefits. One disabled woman with diagnoses of 'arthritis, spinal disease and severe depression', who took her own life, left a suicide note addressed to the Federal Department of Health and Human Services, which said: 'The message that I'm getting is either work or die.' The Reagan administration had reviewed about 1.2 million cases and stopped payment to nearly 500,000 claimants, with 200,000 of those terminations reversed on appeal, until Congress forced a halt to the programme in 1984. State officials throughout the country reported that about one-third of those losing benefits had mental health conditions.

With the close connection between the Reagan and Thatcher administrations, and the influence of the US insurance industry within the DSS – thanks to Peter Lilley's invitation to Unum – it is inconceivable that DSS was unaware of these deaths.

* * *

Just three days before the election, DSS launches the Benefit Integrity Project. The intention is to save £74 million from spending on another benefit, disability living allowance, by examining more than 400,000 existing claimants. This follows a review, ordered by Lilley, which concludes that 27 per cent of claimants had incorrect awards, whether through error or fraud. *Disability Now* magazine will later describe how, as part of the project, DSS will be sending 'benefit spies' into the homes of 250,000 disabled people who claim DLA.[15]

With all attention focused on the election, there is no effective government. A New Labour DSS minister would later say she only learned of the project on 29 May, four weeks after the election.

MPs on the social security sommittee will describe DSS's actions as 'totally unacceptable'.[16]

The decision to go ahead with such a controversial project, just three days before an election, illustrates the cultural problems within DSS. The department's thirst for cuts and hounding disabled people claiming benefits, and for ignoring flaws in its policies and procedures, is becoming clearer. So is the determination that its agenda will not be derailed by something as trivial as democracy.

PART II

1997–2010
DWP, New Labour, and the 'Reckless' Work Capability Assessment

7
Labour's Change of Tone, Atos, and a Failed Rebellion

Tom O'Grady will argue[1] – based on detailed analysis of political debate, media coverage, and public opinion – that Labour's change of tone on social security from the mid-1990s would have a dramatic, lasting impact on welfare reform.

This was a party that had lost four general elections in a row. But after Tony Blair's election as leader in 1994, there was a significant change. From previously supporting social security and its claimants, and the importance of benefits in alleviating poverty, Labour began to join the Conservatives in criticising the system and describing claimants as 'undeserving'. The mainstream press 'followed the same pattern, ramping up criticism during the 1990s'.

Blair feared the public would not believe their shift to the centre ground if they did not take 'unexpected' steps that showed New Labour was different. 'Turning against the welfare system and its users was useful,' says O'Grady, 'because it represented a totemic policy shift in light of the party's past as the founder of much of the welfare state, as well as its image as the party of the poor and downtrodden.' Another factor was the shift in the background of Labour MPs, with increasing numbers of middle-class career politicians and fewer working-class MPs. These new career politicians 'were much more willing to use anti-welfare language'.

These shifts would make it far easier for Labour to introduce its own – damaging and dangerous – welfare reforms.

The May 1997 general election, and the change of government, delays the award of the crucial DSS benefit assessment contract.

Within weeks of the election, some Labour and Liberal Democrat MPs on the left of their parties are raising concerns about the outsourcing plans,[2] with more than 40 – including Dr Roger Berry, Jeremy Corbyn, John McDonnell, and Ken Livingstone – urging the new government to abandon plans to outsource BAMS to the private sector. But incoming ministers almost immediately give their consent to invite tenders.

* * *

18 December 1997. Tony Blair's cabinet meets at 10 Downing Street. On the agenda are proposed cuts to disability benefits, which will help fund increases to health and education.[3] Three days earlier, following a memo leaked to *Channel 4 News*, social security secretary Harriet Harman had been forced to insist in parliament that 'ours is not a cuts-driven agenda' and that 'no one is even talking about taking away benefits from those who need them, disabled or pensioner', although she admits the government is reviewing how to get 'the right support to people who want to work to enable them to do so, and getting the right mix of cash and services to people who cannot work'.[4]

But a 1 December DSS memo, now in the National Archives,[5] suggests that was deeply misleading. It speaks of Harman agreeing to 'a possible "fall back" package of measures that would deliver savings of £1 1/2 Billion'. A series of possible cuts includes options to save more than £1 billion pounds a year from disability living allowance and an option to 'remove through Welfare to Work from IB' 100,000 people, 250,000 people or even 500,000 people. These cuts are proposed even though a later memo[6] admits that incapacity benefit (IB) 'costs and caseload are stable' and there is 'little evidence of incorrectness of award or fraud'. This second memo suggests flaws in the IB system, including 'clear financial incentives to be on IB which can encourage people to present as sick rather than unemployed' while 'many people who could do some work are getting IB' with 'insufficient help and encouragement' to leave the benefit. But it adds: 'Many claimants are too sick and disabled for it to be fair to expect them to work at all, most have passed the test fairly, and most are sufficiently disadvantaged in the labour market that they would find it very hard to get work even if they were strongly motivated to do so.'

Blair insists to his cabinet that the public accept the case for 'fundamental reform of the welfare state, especially when they were confronted with the sheer scale of current expenditure on invalidity and disability benefits'. He tells colleagues the government 'should not yield' and should 'work to communicate the case for change more effectively'.

Political journalist Andrew Rawnsley will later write[7] that Gordon Brown, the chancellor, had asked Harman to find more than £1 billion savings from disability benefits, despite concerns raised by education secretary David Blunkett, himself a disabled person. Blunkett had told Brown that 'deep cuts in support for disabled people who either cannot work or can only find very modestly paid work would make a mockery of our professions on social exclusion and the construction of a more just society'.

Five days after the cabinet meeting, activists from the Disabled People's Direct Action Network, protesting against the proposed cuts, throw red paint over the Downing Street gates.

DSS finally awards the £305 million, five-year assessment contract, in February 1998, to Anglo-French IT services company Sema Group.[8] Sema will be bought out by Schlumberger in 2001 to form SchlumbergerSema, which itself will be taken over by the French company Atos Origin in 2004.

The department believes outsourcing will transfer risk to the private sector, establish clear accountability, and maximise economies of scale. But there is no explicit reference in the contracts to improving the assessment experience for disabled people. DSS reforms have again focused on efficiency and cutting costs. Claimants are seen as numbers, as 'caseload', and not as people whose lives could be placed in jeopardy if the service fails them. And it will.

The government publishes a green paper[9] in which it argues – mirroring Tory language – that fraud is taking money from 'genuine claimants'. The long-delayed paper is authored by welfare reform minister Frank Field, who had promised to deal with what he saw as a 'dependency culture' and had spoken out about benefit fraud.

His green paper calls for fundamental reform of incapacity benefit, arguing that the system 'promotes fraud and deception, not honesty and hard work'. Field will be replaced in the July 1998 reshuffle, but it is growing increasingly difficult to tell the difference between a Tory-run DSS and a department run by New Labour.

Of more than 72,000 claims examined through the Benefit Integrity Project (BIP) – launched under cover of the general election campaign – more than 14,000 were removed completely or reduced, MPs reveal in May 1998.[10]

The social security committee says the project appears to be 'driven by a desire to cut the benefit levels of those reporting severe disability' as it found 'virtually no fraudulent claims'. It says: 'Starting from one position that DLA had a serious problem with fraud, the DSS has moved sharply in barely one year to the position that DLA has virtually no level of fraud whatsoever.' Benefits are often being withdrawn after a single BIP visit, often causing 'extreme distress and anxiety'.

The political context is an administration that Tony Blair has vowed will be a 'Welfare to Work government',[11] with chancellor Gordon Brown pledging to 'rebuild the welfare state around the work ethic'.[12] There are intensified job-search requirements and tougher sanctions for those who do not cooperate, with benefits potentially being removed for six months.[13]

Less than a year after the general election, the New Labour government is already setting about reforming Lilley's all work test. In line with the new 'welfare to work' ethic, it decides it wants to give claimants 'the help and support they need to work in spite of their disabilities'.[14] The new test – which will be named the personal capability assessment – 'will not just determine whether claimants are entitled to benefit, but will also provide additional, constructive information about their capacity for work'.

But the work on reforming incapacity benefit is being driven by civil servants. A memo on 2 April 1998, days earlier, had discussed how those civil servants, including Aylward, wanted to pitch their proposals for a new incapacity assessment to ministers. The memo says they should 'concentrate effort on developing a "capacity for work" assessment'. The next paragraph underlines exactly who is in control:

> My concern would be that putting a specific proposal to Ministers when they have not considered some of the basic issues may create presentational and handling difficulties for us. At the very least Ministers need to be aware that assessing capacity for work is a complex issue which no system in the world has managed to sort out entirely successfully.[15]

The following May, one of New Labour's biggest backbench rebellions sees nearly 70 Labour MPs vote against plans to means-test and tighten access to incapacity benefit in its Welfare Reform and Pensions Bill.[16] The bill introduces the personal capability assessment to replace Lilley's all work test, which Alistair Darling, now secretary of state for social security, says was 'patently subjective' and 'concentrated on what one could not do, rather than on what one could do'. Variations of this phrase will be used again and again by ministers over the next 25 years.

One of the bill's clauses will withdraw entitlement to incapacity benefit from new claimants who have not made enough national insurance contributions in the previous two years. Another will introduce means-testing of incapacity benefit.

Roger Berry, the left-wing MP for Kingswood, who would remain a leading advocate for disability rights in parliament between 1992 and 2010, tells MPs the bill would leave 45,000 disabled people worse off in the first year, rising to 335,000 after ten years, and deny 170,000 people entitlement to any incapacity benefit. Berry refers to Lilley's 1995 reforms, when incapacity benefit was introduced. 'Since then, spending on incapacity benefit has fallen,' he says. 'It is currently about £7.4 billion a year; four years ago, it was nearer £9 billion a year – and it is falling as a result of the latest changes that are feeding through the system. The idea that further cuts to incapacity benefit are necessary because of escalating spending is simply wrong.'

8

The Woodstock Conference, 'Malingering', and an Outlaw Company

There are – so far – four deaths in the 1990s that can be clearly linked to the DSS. There is the sudden death of David Holmes in 1996, Kevin Shields and Dermot Comiskey in early 1997, and then, in November 1998, the death of Timothy Finn. His death – although he was not named – is raised in parliament in March 2000 by the Labour MP for Batley and Spen, Mike Wood.[1]

The debate reveals a few details about Timothy Finn. He was a graduate with a diagnosis of schizophrenia, and his family lived in New Zealand. He had been hospitalised late in 1998. While he was in hospital, his benefits were stopped. He failed to respond to letters from the Benefits Agency. Within months, he had starved to death with just 9p in his pocket. He was found in a sleeping bag in his living room. A note nearby suggested he believed the authorities had killed him.

Records relating to his death in the National Archives were not due to be released until January 2081. They were contained in a number of files I was told would remain closed for decades, with most not to be released until at least 2053. I challenged these decisions under the Freedom of Information Act in November 2022, and after months of discussions between DWP and the National Archives, DWP eventually agreed to release a file containing details of his benefit claim and the inquest into his death, with only minimal redactions.[2]

Timothy Finn lived in Hanging Heaton, just outside Batley, in West Yorkshire. The 48-year-old had been receiving disability benefits for at least ten years, and had been sectioned at least twice.

As he prepares for discharge from his latest stay in a mental health unit, the hospital arranges for an income support claim. He is discharged on 10 February 1998, and applies for incapacity benefit. The Benefits Agency asks for further medical evidence but he fails to provide any. His income support and incapacity benefit continue to be paid – despite his failing to provide the evidence requested – until the middle of April.

In May, his income support claim is closed. The incapacity benefit section sends him four more requests for medical evidence and then closes that claim, too, in June. The Benefits Agency fails to go through the proper all work test procedures.

Finn makes another incapacity benefit claim in August, but again fails to provide any medical evidence when requested. A DSS memo states that he sent a 'confused response', which triggers yet another request for medical evidence. The coroner at his inquest would describe this as 'a plaintive letter'. A DSS officer will tell the inquest that when he first joined the department 20 or 30 years earlier, such a letter would have been dealt with through a visit to the claimant's home. But now, he says, 'people do slip through the net'.

When Finn fails to provide the evidence, his claim is closed on 15 September 'in line with procedures'. His body is found two months later, on 23 November, but he had probably died several weeks earlier. The coroner, Roger Whittaker, will conclude that, in a paranoid delusional state, Finn had 'realised he had no money, he had no food, and he lay down in his sleeping bag and ultimately died of dehydration'. He adds: 'No one, no one, should be allowed to die on their own in such circumstances.'

Whittaker writes what is known as prevention of future deaths reports to the Benefits Agency and the NHS body responsible for his care, after concluding that Finn died due to natural causes 'to which neglect contributed'. He tells the Benefits Agency that he believes its actions were 'a substantial contributory factor in his death'.

The Benefits Agency later claims in a memo that it did not send an officer to check on Finn because 'this would be seen by many customers as an intrusion of privacy' and it 'may be unrealistic' to expect it to involve social services in the lives of its 'customers', although individual members of staff 'do contact Social Services on occasion about clients they have concerns about'.

DSS minister Angela Eagle admits to Mike Wood in March 2000 that it is clear Timothy Finn 'suffered because of a failure by the Department of Social Security and other agencies'. She says new procedures for people with a history of mental distress have been introduced locally and will soon be adopted nationally. This includes advice to claimants to seek advice if they receive letters they don't understand, closer links with social services and mental health services, and 'a new procedure to ensure that no decision will be made to withdraw benefit without the case being referred to a manager'. Despite the new procedures, Timothy Finn's death will not be the last in such circumstances. And Whittaker will not be the last coroner to write a prevention of future deaths letter to the department.

* * *

The name of Unum re-emerges in one of the last Commons debates of 1999, as MPs debate the ordeals of disabled people 'suffering at the hands and sharp practices of some permanent health insurers'.[3]

MPs describe 'evidence of sharp practice' by Unum, which had been involved 'in a series of claims disputes'. One woman with chronic fatigue was followed by a private investigator 'despite overwhelming medical evidence which showed that she was seriously ill'. Labour's Charlotte Atkins says insurance companies 'expanded their operations' after the 1993 budget, when it became clear invalidity benefit would be replaced by incapacity benefit and the amount of money going to sick and disabled people 'would be much reduced'. Many of those companies had been unfairly denying pay-outs, she says.

'Lurid advertisements with graphic tables were designed to shock people into protecting themselves with long-term disability policies,' she says. She refers to Peter Lilley inviting Unum's John LoCascio to work with DSS on the all work test. 'Those tough new tests were fundamental to the savings that [Lilley] hoped to achieve,' she says. 'Dr

LoCascio was therefore helping to validate a scheme that was being exploited by Unum to drum up business in the United Kingdom.'

In March 2001, the National Audit Office (NAO) raises concerns about Labour's new personal capability assessment, which has replaced Lilley's all work test but is based firmly on the same principles.[4] DSS decision-makers can return assessment reports to its contractor Sema if they are not good enough quality. But fewer than 1 per cent are returned, and NAO says staff 'often fail to send back reports that are technically below standard because of the delays it causes, and because they believe the revised report would probably be no better than the first one'.

Government research finds the assessment plagued by many of the same problems as the all work test.[5] It is 'intrinsically stressful'. Some claimants, particularly those with mental distress, find the personal capability assessment 'troubling'. The doctors who carry out the assessments are often described as cold and hostile. These criticisms will persist over the next two decades. The harm, the violence, continues – slowly – to build.

* * *

On 8 June 2001, the day after a general election landslide returns another New Labour government, a new Department for Work and Pensions (DWP) comes into being, cramming together the old Department of Social Security and most of its agencies, significant parts of the Department for Education and Employment, and the Employment Service.

If anything in the New Labour years was to demonstrate how obsessed the department had become with benefit fraud, and its ever-closer links with the private sector, particularly the insurance industry, it was the Woodstock conference.

The conference is held in November 2001 in the eighteenth-century splendour of Blenheim Palace, in Woodstock, Oxfordshire. Its aim is to examine the belief that many claimants of sickness and disability benefits are exaggerating or even faking their symptoms. Many of the academics, historians, civil servants, and medical experts who attend the conference will argue that 'malingering and illness deception' is a lifestyle choice, and that it is widespread.

The conference attracts delegates from the UK and the US, as well as Canada, Australia, and even the Cayman Islands. A book based on the weekend's presentations, published two years later, titled *Malingering and Illness Deception*, will be co-edited by psychologists Peter Halligan (who would later become the government's chief scientific adviser for Wales), Christopher Bass, and David Oakley.[6] It will acknowledge the conference 'would not have been possible had it not been for the enthusiastic support of Professor Mansel Aylward and funding from the Department for Work and Pensions'.

Despite his wish in later years to downplay his role, a photograph of the 30-odd participants, proudly posing on the palace steps, shows Aylward at the centre of the front row. He is joined by Unum's Dr John LoCascio and both make significant contributions, as does Professor Gordon Waddell, who will also play a key part in furthering DWP's agenda.

When I ask Aylward about the conference, 20 years later, he appears embarrassed. He suggests it was driven by Halligan and Cardiff University, where Halligan was based. Aylward initially claims it was not funded by DWP, until I tell him I have seen proof it was (it is mentioned in the acknowledgements of the book). And when I suggest it was regrettable that DWP sponsored a conference titled 'Malingering and Illness Deception', he says: 'Well, the conference was exceptionally good because it didn't talk about malingering.'

Despite this claim, the book, which is based on presentations made at the conference, includes 43 mentions of the word 'malinger', 1,707 of 'malingering', 80 of 'malingerer', and 121 of 'malingerers'.

Aylward claims he himself has never used the word 'malingerer', but it is mentioned several times in his Woodstock paper,[7] and in another influential article he co-wrote.[8] He says he now regrets attending the conference.

What is striking about the Woodstock papers later published by Oxford University Press is the assumption held by many delegates that widespread 'malingering and illness deception' exists among claimants of disability benefits. Yet nowhere among its 27 chapters is there any suggestion of research proving the existence of widespread fakery and fraud. No one sensible would deny there is a – probably very small – minority of people who exaggerate or even invent an impairment because they prefer not to work. To suggest otherwise would be like pretending there is no such thing as theft, violence, or dishonesty. But the assumption of most of the delegates, clearly supported by those at the heart of the new DWP, is that this is a major problem, and that it demands significant tightening of assessment procedures. This belief was a convenient one for DWP and the government, with their cost-cutting agenda, but many of the delegates clearly believed in this argument, despite the lack of hard evidence.

The opening paper, by Halligan, Bass, and Oakley, makes sweeping assumptions, but with little evidence. They talk of 'illness behaviours' and 'illness deception'. Their excuse for having no proof of widespread deception is that 'prevalence rates for malingering are under-investigated'. They repeatedly quote research that relies on 'anecdotal evidence', and talk of 'estimates of the prevalence of malingering and symptom exaggeration'.

Halligan, Bass, and Oakley make much of the rising number of incapacity benefit claimants over the previous 30 years, but ignore the explanations for large parts of that increase, repeatedly put forward by politicians and researchers.

One delegate, lawyer Michael Jones, provides some balance,[9] and points out that DSS (now DWP) 'has found very little evidence of malingering'. In fact, a 2001 DWP review of a random sample of 1,401 incapacity benefit claimants found just three cases of confirmed fraud, he says, and estimated the percentage of fraudulent cases was less than 0.5 per cent.

Mansel Aylward had been at the heart of DSS for a decade. He and LoCascio had worked increasingly closely together since Peter Lilley appealed for insurance industry expertise in July 1992, and they co-authored a paper in 1995 which attempted to demonstrate the importance of what they call disability assessment medicine.[10]

Aylward's paper discusses the origins of disability assessment medicine. He writes about his work with LoCascio and their concern about the 'indiscriminate acceptance of subjective health complaints' by the medical profession, 'ill-defined medical conditions', and the 'growing numbers of syndromes and disorders defined in terms of symptoms rather than pathology'. He appears to be suggesting that many of the symptoms and conditions that the medical profession doesn't yet understand are likely to be manifestations of 'malingering' and that symptoms of pain, fatigue, and mental distress are 'subjective'. He argues for the application of a so-called 'biopsychosocial model', in which a claimant's 'attitudes and beliefs' about their health problems provide a 'better understanding' of their 'illness behaviours'.

This unevidenced biopsychosocial model, and its adoption by DWP, will play a significant role in causing harm to claimants, and will remain at the centre of the department's system for assessing benefit claims. Aylward argues that what he calls 'illness behaviours' may be 'driven by the subject's choice and intent'. This provides a 'formidable barrier' to the healthcare professional carrying out an assessment 'when deception is strongly suspected'. He calls for the 'sensitivities and ambiguities surrounding the attribution of malingering and illness deception' to be 'robustly confronted and resolved'.

A recording unearthed by the BBC for a radio documentary broadcast in 2023[11] has Aylward explaining that it was people's beliefs that stopped them working, a theory which sat at the centre of his all work test. 'It was because of their beliefs and their attitudes,' he says, '... and we tackled those'.

In his paper,[12] Unum's LoCascio supports calls for 'preventive measures' that would 'change the payoff matrix in such a way that it discourages malingering'. In other words, cut the generosity of incapacity benefits. This should be done through 'legislation, regulation, and the design of innovative commercial products'. Which of course will benefit Unum.

But for all the exasperation of the authors of the *Malingering and Illness Deception* papers, there is almost no hard evidence of significant levels of disability benefit fraud. Instead, there is significant evidence of guesswork and a discriminatory attitude among many of them. Of even more concern is that this approach has become ingrained right at the heart of the DSS and will help set the harshest of tones for the new Department for Work and Pensions.

Meanwhile, Unum's practices in the US are beginning to cause concern. NBC[13] and CBS[14] both air documentaries detailing allegations about Unum's behaviour, in October and November 2002. Unum staff processing private insurance claims are said to be pressured by managers to deny valid claims, with bonuses awarded to some managers who have denied particularly large claims. Two years later, Unum settles a multi-state legal case, which identifies the company's use of medically trained staff to deny, terminate, or reduce insurance payments to disabled people.[15] In 2005, California's insurance commissioner will describe Unum as 'an outlaw company' which 'for years has operated in an illegal fashion', after charging it with more than 25 violations of state law.[16]

This is the company that has worked its way into the heart of the UK government, and whose advice – particularly through LoCascio – has become central to reforming the assessment processes that will determine whether disabled people receive the support they need.

Back in the UK, Unum continues to lobby for a harsher incapacity benefit system. In December, it submits a memo to the Commons work and pensions committee.[17] The memo makes clear Unum's size and influence. In the UK it holds income protection insurance policies for more than 737,000 individuals and pays about £116 million a year in benefits to disabled people. But Unum wants to expand. It tells the committee that the current social security and tax systems are 'overly complex' and 'provide strong disincentives for disabled people to look for work'. It argues that there is a 'strong case' for fundamental reform of the incapacity benefit system, adding: 'The Government must ensure both that work always pays more than benefits, and more importantly that it is clearly seen to do so.' It is arguing for substantial cuts to benefits.

It says incapacity benefit 'should be retained for those disabled people who are genuinely incapable of undertaking any work whatsoever', while the others 'should be transferred to a form of Job Seekers Allowance (JSA) which is sufficiently flexible to recognise that they have limited capacity to work'. It is a blueprint for a system that the New Labour government will introduce less than six years later.

We now begin to enter the years where records have yet to be released under the National Archives 20-year rule, so we know less about what was going on within DWP, and what civil servants were saying to each other and to ministers and the private sector about disability benefit reform.

But public documents, academic research, and parliamentary debates show the direction of policy was unchanged, and that the private sector was slowly tightening its grip on DWP and the assessment process.

By now, says Tom O'Grady,[18] 'neither politicians nor newspapers were speaking in positive terms about the welfare system, and voters could not help but notice'. The years of pressure from politicians and the media to clamp down on social security spending – influenced by the DSS/DWP, with the insurance industry pulling its strings – are having an impact. The public are steadily turning against claimants, particularly those receiving disability benefits. Further reform, further tightening of eligibility, further cuts, are becoming ever more possible.

Meanwhile, Unum has been preparing another attempt at securing academic respectability for its attack on the benefits system. In May 2004, it announces a new five-year partnership with Cardiff University that aims to explore 'why some people respond differently to the same disease' and why the same condition 'renders some people unable to work while others continue'.[19] Unum has funded the £1.66 million research contract for the new UnumProvident Centre for Psychosocial and Disability Research in the university's School of Psychology. The aim is for the centre to become 'a recognised world-class research centre and resource for psychosocial and disability research'.

The academic from the university's psychology department who 'forged' the partnership with Unum, and is its new associate director, says: 'Hopefully within five years, the work will bring about a significant re-orientation in current medical practise in the UK whereby "enablement" rather than disability, will be the positive focus and goal for those involved in managing disability and those affected by unexplained symptoms.' The academic is Professor Peter Halligan, the driving force behind the 2001 Woodstock event and co-editor of *Malingering and Illness Deception*.

When the centre opens two months later, the close relationships with DWP, and with MPs, are clear. Archy Kirkwood, the Liberal Democrat MP who now chairs the Commons work and pensions committee, is there, and work and pensions minister Malcolm Wicks delivers a speech. Mansel Aylward, by now a professor, is appointed the centre's director after retiring as DWP's chief medical officer. He will be replaced at DWP in June 2005 by Dr Bill Gunnyeon, who moves from the outsourcing giant Capita, which will itself later secure a significant benefits assessment contract, and had bid unsuccessfully for the assessment contract awarded to Sema in 1998.[20] Writing later about the launch in the centre's first newsletter[21] is Unum director Dr Peter Dewis, who worked alongside Aylward for many years at DWP.

If there is any doubt about Unum's motives, the proof comes the following year in one of its 'Group Income Protection' leaflets,[22] in which Michael O'Donnell, Unum's chief medical officer, says: 'We know that our views and understanding are not yet in the mainstream of doctors' thinking, but Government Policy is moving in the same direction, to a large extent being driven by our thinking and that of our close associates, both in the UK and overseas.'

Aylward will tell me in 2023 that he had no problem working with Unum at the Cardiff centre, but he claims he didn't learn much from them. Instead, he says: 'I learned a lot of what not to do. I learned a lot of what they did in America. Which we don't [do in the UK]. But other than that, you know, it was a passing fancy.' He insists he had no idea that Unum was lobbying parliament and the government for stricter benefit eligibility. 'I didn't know that,' he says. 'I swear on the Bible I didn't know that. Never mentioned to me at all. By any party.'

As Unum lobbies for further and tougher reform of incapacity benefits, it is doing so in lockstep with DWP, despite Aylward's protestations. 'The Scientific and Conceptual Basis of Incapacity Benefits', by Gordon Waddell and Mansel Aylward,[23] both now at Unum's centre in Cardiff, argues for the application of the biopsychosocial model of disability. It is published by DWP in October 2005 and takes on the arguments discussed at Woodstock, pushing the Unum line that it is not their impairments or the barriers that disabled people face in society that prevent them working, but their own faults, flaws, and unwillingness to work. Their book provides, they say, 'a scientific evidence base for reform'.

The book, one researcher will say later,[24] provides 'the unacknowledged intellectual framework' for the government's welfare reform bill, which will be published the following year. That bill will – by replacing the personal capability assessment and incapacity benefit with the work capability assessment and employment and support allowance – set the country even further along the path that will lead to countless deaths of disabled people.

9
A Groundswell of Unease

By 2005, the New Labour government and DWP are approaching the final stages of their major reform of incapacity benefits. In May, Anne McGuire is appointed minister for disabled people. Although not responsible for incapacity benefit reform, she works on the plans with Margaret Hodge, the minister for work, and her successor, Jim Murphy, who becomes minister for employment and welfare reform in May 2006.

'We knew there had to be changes,' McGuire tells me years later. 'The disability lobby knew there had to be changes. Even if, you know, they didn't necessarily like all aspects of the outcomes, they were certainly engaged in those discussions.'

She cannot remember being told by DWP civil servants of any historic deaths linked to the all work test. 'I certainly don't recollect anything like that … I mean, there are so many bits of paper passed to you, but I would've remembered something like that.' The department, it seems, has filed away those deaths previously linked to its assessment regimes.

From November 2005 until June 2007, DWP is led by John Hutton. He will later argue[1] that having so many people on incapacity benefits was 'a total failure of the welfare state' and in exchange for 'providing more help' into work, claimants had 'resulting responsibilities' to 'do everything they could themselves to get back into work.' He claimed 'the vast majority' of those on incapacity benefit 'wanted some help to get back into work.' There appears to be no evidence for this claim. Most of those on incapacity benefit were not fit for work and knew they were not fit for work, and wanted to be left alone by DWP. DWP's own figures in 2023[2] found the proportion of economically inactive disabled people who wanted a job in 2021–22 was just 22 per cent.

DWP sets up numerous working groups to fine-tune its plans. There are representatives of the disability charities, the insurance industry (including Unum and Atos), and the Faculty of Occupational Medicine, which is right at the heart of the supposed science of disability assessment medicine.

One of the members of the mental health technical working group is Professor Geoff Shepherd, a clinical psychologist and a senior policy adviser at the Sainsbury Centre for Mental Health. He will eventually resign from the working group.

He told me years later that 'everybody thought' the new work capability assessment (WCA) would harm claimants. 'It was barn door obvious it was never going to work, and it was always going to be very stressful for people,' he said. His impression, from the beginning, is that DWP is insistent and reckless about its direction.

He also realises the department is 'in bed with Atos', which had won a £500 million, five-year contract to carry out the assessments for incapacity benefit in 2005 and would secure a further three-year extension in 2010. The department is 'wedded to the idea that this was the way assessments had always been done'.

'They were prepared to listen to comments about the wording of questions and the content of questions, but to my mind that really just misses the point,' he told me.

Hutton told the BBC in 2023 that he had 'no knowledge, none whatsoever' of concerns raised by the mental health technical working group, which called on DWP to delay its reforms. 'I never received that advice,' he would say. McGuire also says she was not made aware of the working group's concerns.

Shepherd said the focus of the WCA was to cut costs.

> It is fair to say, I think, it is a reckless process because it wasn't thought through. The purpose really wasn't to do an assessment of people with mental health and other problems to see whether they were capable of work or not. The purpose was to save money and chase them back into work and save money on the welfare budget.

Then he reconsiders the word 'reckless' and tells me: 'I don't think they were reckless at all, they were ruthless.'

> I have absolutely no doubt that it could have been predicted that the process was going to be very distressing, very stressful, because it is so flawed. The fact that the process is so bad makes it stressful, because it is a bit like Russian roulette: you don't know if there is a bullet in the chamber or not … I can very easily believe that it would damage people's mental health, at least in the short term, and I can believe that it might lead to suicide.

Anne McGuire – now Dame Anne McGuire – believes there were 'certain elements' within DWP that were a 'hangover' from the 1980s and the 1990s, when the aim had not always been to act in claimants' best interests. She contrasts that with the Office for Disability Issues, set up under Labour within DWP, which she had hoped would be 'the catalyst to trying to change some attitudes within the organisation' and which allowed her to work with ministers across government on a 'positive' disability rights agenda.

She accepts that the insurance companies were 'starting to make inroads' within DWP, and she adds:

> We inherited a department that culturally was maybe in a different place than where we would want it to be, certainly given our agenda for improving the lives of disabled people. I would hope that, after the early 2000s, we were trying successfully, or at least semi-successfully, to turn the ship around and to get a far more positive outlook.

Perhaps some of her ministerial colleagues had a different perspective.

In January 2006, Hutton publishes a long-delayed green paper, 'A New Deal for Welfare',[3] which introduces employment and support allowance, the proposed replacement for incapacity benefit. 'After two years on incapacity benefits, a person is more likely to die or retire than to find a new job,' says Hutton. 'It is not acceptable to write off millions of people in this way … Benefits trap people into a lifetime of dependency.'

The aspiration, he says, is to 'reduce the number of incapacity benefits claimants by one million over the course of a decade'. It is a staggering target. Under the new system, most people on the new benefit will have to take part in job-related interviews, agree an action plan and take part in 'work-related activity', or face having their benefits cut. Only those claimants with 'the most severe health conditions or disabilities' will not face any conditions.

The following month, Citizens Advice Bureau will publish a worrying report,[4] warning that the existing assessment system is 'not working satisfactorily' – with frequent complaints about the conduct of face-to-face assessments – and that 'too often evidence from the Atos Origin doctor is preferred over other evidence supplied by practitioners who are more familiar with the applicant's condition', and particularly highlighting the 'injustice' faced by people with mental health problems, who 'face real difficulties receiving and retaining the benefits to which they are entitled'.

On the same day the green paper is published, the BBC launches a new TV series, *On the Fiddle*, which aims to spotlight the tiny minority of people who claim incapacity benefit fraudulently. It is the first in a series of programmes – documentary is too generous a word – that will support the Labour and subsequent Tory-led governments in their attacks on disabled people claiming benefits. They will contribute significantly to the hostile environment – and hate crime – many of them face in their daily lives.

Alongside the green paper, just three months after he and Mansel Aylward published 'The Scientific and Conceptual Basis of Incapacity Benefits', Gordon Waddell – still with the Unum research centre – publishes another controversial document, this time with occupational health expert Kim Burton. 'Is Work Good for Your Health and Well-being?'[5] has been commissioned by DWP and argues that work 'is generally good for physical and mental health and well-being'. It is exactly the message DWP and ministers want to push, and it provides crucial (and lasting) academic cover for a fresh push to force disabled people off out-of-work benefits.

Only a few voices warn of the damage that will be done. Among them is author and academic Alison Ravetz, who publishes a paper[6] warning of the significant stress that will be caused to those forced into the job market. She highlights the lack of supporting evidence for claims made in the green paper and DWP reports, which fail to accept the reality of disabled people's lives.

She concludes:

> … what might be expected is a slowly accumulating number of bad decisions and blatantly scandalous cases, eventually giving rise to a groundswell of unease … In the long run, this reform will stand or fall by the correctness of its belief that two thirds of all claimants are well enough to compete as jobseekers in the labour market. If this is wrong, the cost to society of a system that forces people into jobs they cannot sustain, on threat of penury, might well outweigh any financial savings; while the cost, in stress, to those people and their families will be incalculable.

Ravetz's words, and her warning of slow violence, will prove chillingly accurate.

The following year, DWP publishes a report by David Freud,[7] an investment banker commissioned to review the government's Welfare to Work programme, who will later switch sides and become a Tory peer and DWP minister. Freud concludes that, if the government wants to achieve its target of 80 per cent of the working-age population in employment, it will need to reduce the number claiming incapacity benefits from 2.68 million to 1.68 million.

He recommends 'increasing' the conditions expected of those on 'inactive' benefits like incapacity benefit. He says those on the new employment and support allowance (ESA) should have monthly interviews 'with an associated requirement to engage in activity that will prepare them for work', although he says there will need to be 'sensitivity' and 'safeguards' when applying sanctions to people with mental health conditions, while the strict conditions should not apply to claimants with 'the most severe disabilities and health conditions'.

In May 2007, Labour's package of reforms, including the introduction of ESA and the new work capability assessment, receives royal assent as the Welfare Reform Act.[8] As Unum had lobbied for, at least as far back as 2002, there will be three new groups. Some will be found fit for work, and will have to either find work or claim the mainstream jobseeker's allowance (JSA). Another group will be seen as having limited capability for work, with conditions placed upon the continued payment of a more generous allowance than JSA. The final group, the 'support group', will be – the government hopes – a small number of those found to have limited capability for both work and work-related activity, who will therefore have no conditions placed upon them. Crucially, not just doctors but other healthcare professionals – nurses, paramedics, and even occupational therapists – will carry out the new assessments.

In November, Labour announces details of the new work capability assessment. The aim, according to Peter Hain, Hutton's replacement as work and pensions secretary, is for half of new claimants to be found fit for work. It will be introduced for new claimants in October 2008.

Hain is slightly more circumspect in the DWP press release[9] than in his media interviews, saying: 'We know that many people want to work – work is good for you and your long-term well-being and we don't think it's right that in the past people were effectively written off. We want to work with people to get them back into jobs and help them stay there.'

But the hostility is ratcheted up in a *Daily Mirror* interview.[10] 'In the past, people going on IB were written off, more likely to reach retirement age or die than work again,' Hain says. 'At its height this cost £15 billion a year, embedding the sick-note into the British economy. We must rip up sick-note Britain.'

The Guardian calls on Matthew Elliott, from the Taxpayers' Alliance, to add an extra dose of scrounger rhetoric: 'Many incapacity claimants are clearly taking advantage of the good nature of their GPs,' he says. 'There is a huge difference between not being able to work and not feeling like working.'[11]

The following February, Freud claims in an interview with *The Telegraph*[12] that fewer than a third of the 2.7 million people on incapacity benefit are legitimate claimants. He provides no evidence for this, and claims the system 'sends 2.64 million people into a form of economic house arrest and encourages them to stay at home and watch daytime TV'.

Yet another new work and pensions secretary, James Purnell, warns that DWP advisers will be given more powers to impose sanctions.[13] Jobcentre Plus chief executive Lesley Strathie will lead a review that includes looking at sanctions for those 'playing the system'. The new sanctions will 'tackle those people who can work and choose not to,' says Purnell.

In April 2008, he continues the attack, telling the *Liverpool Echo*[14] the government wants to clamp down on benefit cheats. 'People who scrounge from the system take money away from legitimate [IB] claimants. Clearly we want to stop that,' he says.

Employment and support allowance (ESA) – and, alongside it, the work capability assessment and a stricter regime of conditions – is introduced for new claimants in October 2008. For the moment, those already claiming incapacity benefit are left alone, but the programme to reassess them is on the horizon.

There is little opposition. *The Guardian* applauds Purnell[15] for pointing out that 'the more cynical path would actually be to leave the system as it is', where 'the 2.7m people currently on IB would be kept conveniently apart from official unemployment statistics', a 'sleight of hand' that was 'devised by the Tories in the 1990s', and which 'all but guaranteed that victims of 1980s deindustrialisation would become reliant on long-term welfare'. This is an odd reading of Peter Lilley's incapacity benefit reforms, which were aimed at cutting costs and reducing the number of claimants.

The following October, at her party conference, shadow work and pensions secretary Theresa May promises that a Conservative government would force hundreds of thousands of claimants off incapacity benefits. 'When we retest all the existing claimants of IB,' she says, 'those who are found to be fit for work will be moved onto JSA and have their benefits cut accordingly.'

Steve Donnison, co-founder of the Benefits and Work website, says the party seems to be 'involved in a bidding war with Labour to see who can stir up the most prejudice against sick and disabled claimants'.[16] 'Whoever gets in,' he says, 'it looks like we're in for years of hasty, unreliable medical assessments and huge quantities of money being poured into the private sector to push sick and disabled people into short-term, insecure work which will probably make them so ill they'll then have no trouble qualifying for ESA.'

Meanwhile, the *Daily Express* publishes a story[17] – one of many similar attacks over the next few years – that attempts to whip up public anger with claimants of incapacity benefit. It incorrectly reports the results of early DWP statistics on the new ESA, claiming they show that 75 per cent of existing claimants of incapacity benefit are 'faking'.

In fact, the first published ESA statistics show only about 39 per cent of new claimants have been found fit for work. Another 42 per cent stopped claiming benefits before the assessment process was completed (often because they had recovered from a short-term health condition).[18] Crucially, the claimants who are being tested are an entirely different group than those already receiving incapacity benefit, many of whom have been doing so for many years because of long-term impairments. It is a theme that will be repeated countless times over the next decade: stirring up antagonism among the public, scapegoating disabled people, creating a climate of fear among claimants, and providing cover for politicians. The consequences will be long-lasting and fatal.

10
The Death of Stephen Carré

January 2010. The front door of 3 Coral Close is hidden behind a hedge at the end of the cul-de-sac. It is a wide road, but number 3 is squashed into a corner, a garage directly in front of it.

Stephen's girlfriend hadn't seen Stephen for about ten days. This wasn't unheard of, but she was concerned enough to want to check he was OK. He hadn't been answering the phone. The downstairs curtains were drawn, as always. She rang the bell, called out his name, but there was no answer. She tried the handle. It was unlocked, and she pulled the handle down and pushed open the door.

> Police were called to a house in Coral Close, Eaton Bray, at lunchtime on Monday, January 18, after the body of a man was found.
>
> Officers went to the scene after receiving a call from a visitor to the property.
>
> It is not believed that there are any suspicious circumstances regarding the death.
>
> A post mortem and inquest will be held at a later date, once the next of kin have been informed.
>
> Update:
> An inquest was today opened following the death of 41-year-old villager Stephen Carre, who died at his home on Monday 18th January … The inquest has been adjourned and will be resumed at a later date. (www.eatonbray.com)

'Stephen was my baby brother,' Sarah Carré tells me years later. 'As is the way with most baby brothers, he was a pain in the butt, but I loved him, even when we were fighting.' She remembers a teacher running to fetch her at school because Stephen was inconsolable and wanted his big sister. 'He threw himself into my arms, just sobbing.' It took a few minutes before he told her he was upset because he had chewing gum in his hair.

'He was a really cute kid, with blonde hair, and brown eyes, which went so well with his tan that he gained from spending most days on the beach in Malta. It was hardly surprising that he melted hearts.'

Stephen had been born on 11 January 1969 at a British military hospital in West Germany, where his father Peter was stationed in the army. He was educated at British forces schools in Germany and Malta before his parents split up, and later attended school in Lincolnshire.

Stephen was not shy with adults. 'He was always able to hold a sensible conversation, even from a very early age, and was inquisitive, so asked questions, usually pertinent ones, and he usually understood the answers he was given,' says Peter. He was given a computer, a Sinclair Spectrum, and quickly learned how to program it. Once he'd set his mind to something, he was single-minded. He played hockey at school and eventually represented the county. He later took up climbing and became a qualified climbing and ice climbing instructor.

His sister remembers Stephen as much more of a 'people person' than she was, so they rarely played together. When they did, they would often end up fighting. She remembers long car journeys around Europe, with back seat disagreements that were annoying at the time but are precious memories now. 'I went to boarding school when I was nine, so I only saw him during the school holidays. I would get more and more excited towards the end of term because I would be seeing him.' When they eventually moved to England, they would each spend part of the holidays with each parent, and so spent even less time together.

Hormones hit him hard in his teens and he turned into a stroppy and troubled teenager. Sarah says now that she believes her brother was autistic. She rebelled as a teenager, left home at 16 and lost touch with Stephen for several years because she couldn't phone the house in case their mother answered.

While he is at university in York, Sarah visits her brother with their mother a few days before Christmas. He had turned, she says, into 'a really nice man'. They go Christmas shopping and he asks her to choose a present. She wants a teddy bear, thinking he will buy her a cheap £5 bear from Woolworths. They don't have any, so they continue searching until they see a large, beautiful bear sat high up on a shelf. The shopkeeper brings it down, and tells them it is £120. She hands it back, but Stephen says, no, you can have him. 'That bear is still one of my most treasured possessions, not because he was so expensive, but because Stephen had been so generous and kind. That day – the whole day – was probably the day that I treasured most with my brother.'

After university, Stephen joins the civil service, specialising in IT, and then works for electronics and communications companies including Cisco and Ericsson. He helps write and maintain the billing programs for mobile phones. He has two passports, because he works both in Israel and Palestine. He works all over the world, frequently in remote areas, and his family will often not hear from him for months. His skills are greatly in demand within the industry.

'As an adult, away from his work environment, he found it difficult to relate to people in general and became quite introverted,' his father remembers. His step-mother, Frances, 'could always pull him out of himself after a while, as could his step-sister Fiona, with whom he got on very well'. But, says Peter, 'he had to know someone for a while before he could hold a real conversation'.

By the time he is in his 30s, he is living in Milton Keynes in a tiny flat, working ridiculous hours. 'I picked up that he wasn't very happy, despite his many interests,' says Sarah. He starts dating his sister's lodger, but it doesn't last long. 'My lodger was the type that needed someone to make her do the running, whereas Stephen wanted to treat her like royalty,' says Sarah. He was devastated when it ended, and when she talked to her brother, she found out that all he wanted was a partner and children. 'He desperately wanted his own family,' she says.

Stephen meets Glenda, who was divorced, in about 1999. Sarah was thrilled to hear Glenda was pregnant, and then that she had had a girl. 'My mother and I made the journey down to see them, and I fell head over heels with my niece. It was obvious that Stephen was besotted with her. It was the happiest that I'd seen him.'

They have a son soon afterwards, Matthew, but Glenda has taken a dislike to Sarah, so she can no longer visit her brother and his new family. Stephen and Glenda split up soon after Matthew is born. After they separate, he misses his children a great deal, says Peter. He buys a house in Eaton Bray, a small village in Bedfordshire, while Glenda and the children continue to live nearby.

In June 2007, Stephen suddenly stops working as a telecommunications consultant. He will not talk to anyone. He won't answer the door or the phone. Peter and Frances drive to see him and put a note through his letterbox, but he never replies. For a while they lose touch.

Glenda has moved north to be near her parents. By now, says Peter, he was not coping well and could not make the journey to Cheshire to visit. Sarah tries to get in touch, but Stephen cannot talk about his depression.

Early in 2009, his father tries again to contact his son. Stephen puts the phone down when he hears his father's voice. Peter calls again. His son is in tears. Peter and Frances drive down to see him from their home in Ipswich. Stephen is living in one room on the ground floor. Everything he needs is piled around him. By now he has exhausted his savings, and Peter eventually persuades him to apply for out-of-work benefits. He is clearly unable to work, and has been receiving treatment from his GP, a community psychiatric nurse, and a consultant psychiatrist.

Stephen begins his claim for the new employment and support allowance (ESA) in April 2009. Peter and Frances have been paying his mortgage. For the first three months, he receives a small weekly payment of just over £60 while he waits for DWP's contractor, Atos, to assess his ability to work.

He fills out an ESA50 questionnaire, which is supposed to demonstrate his capability for work. He says he is taking medication for depression and for sleeping problems, and he provides contact details for both his GP and the specialists at the local mental health trust.

Although many of the boxes on the form – including the 'physical functions' section – are ticked 'no', there are also areas of his life where he has significant concerns. He often cannot concentrate on his daily routines, he needs reminding to take his medication, and he 'usually' has difficulties finishing routine daily jobs. 'Washing up sits for days before getting done,' he writes. 'Some weeks don't shop at all. Some days, don't cook or eat at all. Lack of motivation and enthusiasm.' He often cannot cope with unexpected small changes to his routine. 'Known changes – if a bad day, won't answer door or phone even if expected. Won't ever answer door or phone if not expected.'

When asked if the thought of meeting new people or going to new places makes him anxious or scared, he says: 'Don't feel inclined to go out.' Asked if he gets so upset by 'little things or by the way other people behave that it affects your daily routine', he answers yes, and adds: 'If persistent callers, either phone or to house, I end up shouting and swearing at phone/door.'

He is given a date of 25 July for his assessment, on the sixth floor of a grim office block in the centre of Luton. 'He couldn't go anywhere on his own for the first time,' Peter would say later. He drives his son to the assessment centre in Luton at least twice, until he is comfortable going there on his own. 'He did want to go back to work,' said Peter, 'he just couldn't manage it. Even though he'd lived [in the area] for years, he wouldn't go anywhere that he wasn't familiar with.'

Stephen tells the doctor at the assessment that his mental distress was caused by relationship problems and 'work related stress', and that he left his job because of his mental health. He describes shutting himself away from society for two years and says he had not sought help until he visited his GP in February 2009. He has been attending a psychiatric outpatient clinic, and speaks of mood changes, loss of interest, and a lack of motivation. He also tells the doctor he wakes at about 4am 'or earlier' and does not do any housework. He appears to spend much of his time reading novels. He is thinking of retraining as he had been advised by his GP and psychiatrist not to go back to his previous job, and has an appointment to see the government work programme contractor Shaw Trust.

But in his assessment report, the Atos doctor says Stephen did not look tired, 'did not appear to be trembling' or sweating and was 'able to sit still during the interview'. He concludes that Stephen is 'unlikely to have a significant level of disability affecting their ability to cope with change, get to familiar places, get to unfamiliar places and cope with social situations'. He also concludes that there is no evidence to suggest Stephen's depression 'is uncontrolled, uncontrollable or life threatening or that it poses a substantial risk to anyone' and that he 'may return to work in the shorter term'. The report is completed by the doctor on 2 August, eight days after the assessment.

As a result of the report, he is told in September that DWP has found him fit for work. On every one of the 21 'activities' the doctor assessed him on, he has been given a zero score. The information Stephen receives from DWP is littered with errors. It says he is not interested in housing benefit and council tax benefit, although he is. It says he is not receiving any specialist treatment. But he is. It says he has earned more than £16,000 that year. But he hasn't worked since June 2007. The assessment report is dated 2 July 2009, although Stephen was assessed on 25 July.

Stephen appeals against the decision. He tells DWP the medical assessment 'bears no relation to the medical I had' and points out the mistake with the dates. He says the assessment 'disagrees wildly' with the opinion of his GP, his community psychiatric nurse, the mental health trust, and his consultant psychiatrist.

'He was always reluctant to talk about the medical assessment afterwards,' says Peter, 'but anyone with a modicum of intelligence could have seen immediately that Stephen was incapable of normal social intercourse and how he could possibly have been scored at zero after his assessment – which meant he was found fit for work – is totally beyond me.' His father last sees Stephen two days before Christmas.

Early in the new year, on 12 January, the Luton Benefit Delivery Centre writes to Stephen again, to inform him of the result of his appeal. In the latest of a string of errors, the last paragraph of the decision notice refers to Stephen as 'Mr Paul David Carter'. It says he failed to provide any additional medical evidence, or indicate which scores he disagreed with. There had been no indication on the appeal form that a claimant should provide additional evidence, or that he needed to highlight which parts he disagreed with. The form confirms the original decision: he is fit for work and cannot receive ESA.

He submits an appeal to the tribunal almost immediately. By the time his appeal papers arrive at 3 Coral Close, Stephen has taken his own life.

When they visit the house later, Stephen's parents see he had recently been shopping; there is food in the fridge, and he had bought a new tea-towel.

His sister hears the news on 18 January, the day Stephen's body is found. She is working as a countryside ranger and has been on a speedboat course and so has not had her phone with her all day. She sees multiple missed calls from her mother and when she calls her back, her mum tells her: 'Stephen's dead.'

'I went cold from my head to my toes, my brain refusing to accept what she was saying,' Sarah told me. 'Then again when she said that it was suicide. I don't think I warmed up for months. I just felt this fury, disbelief, denial, and an absolute grinding guilt that I hadn't been able to protect my baby brother the way that I had done when we were children. Even though he and I had spent so little of our lives together in a real sense, I'd always held onto the fact that he was out there, somewhere, and now he wasn't. I still feel that lack every day.'

Days before Stephen's death, government figures show only a small proportion of people applying for ESA are being found not fit for work.[1] The Labour government claims the figures show that 'thousands of people are now moving towards work rather than being left to claim sickness benefit'. Of the 326,500 people who completed new claims between October 2008 and May 2009, only about 59,000 (18 per cent) have been found eligible for ESA. Of these, only about

18,000 (5.5 per cent) are placed in the support group, for those who do not have to take part in work-related activity.

The years of negative attacks on the system and on claimants have had their effect. 'The constraint on radical welfare reform from public opinion had shifted, making it politically feasible,' Tom O'Grady will write later.[2] Labour's own attacks on the system will provide 'political cover' for the next government. 'By 2010 the three main British parties were all competing with each other to be tough on welfare. There was consensus, and this enabled change.' O'Grady says it took just 15 years to go from only 25 per cent of the British public believing in 1994 that unemployment benefits were too high and discouraged work to 62 per cent in 2008. It is fertile territory for what will come next.

* * *

March 2010. About 18 months after its introduction, DWP publishes an internal review of the work capability assessment (WCA),[3] based on the first few thousand ESA claimants. The review concludes that the test 'is accurately identifying individuals' capability for work', although it recommends refinements.

It calls for changes in areas where the assessment 'could be amended to better account for adaptation', or how disabled people adapt to their impairments. The recommendations – described by the Benefits and Work website as 'ugly plans'[4] – are published weeks before the general election. Benefits and Work says the changes will make it harder to claim ESA.

DWP publishes *Building Bridges to Work*,[5] which speaks of rolling out the WCA to long-term claimants of incapacity benefit to – once again – 'look at what they can do, not just what they can't do'. A Labour government – if re-elected – will assess 10,000 people on incapacity benefit a week, starting with trials in October 2010, with 'an ambitious timetable to abolish old style incapacity benefits by 2014'. The WCA, the paper says, 'is rightly assessing more people as fit for work'.

Meanwhile, a report from Citizens Advice[6] is raising grave concerns about the WCA. *Not Working* includes a string of cases in which medical examiners have carried out hurried medicals, missed vital details, made 'unjustifiable assumptions', or failed to place enough emphasis on the impact of mental distress on people's ability to work. It says Citizens Advice staff have reported 'high numbers' of 'seriously ill and disabled people' found fit for work after undergoing the assessment.

The inquest into Stephen Carré's death takes place two months after his death. The coroner, Tom Osborne, hears from Stephen's GP and his psychiatrist. They make it clear that they had not been asked for their opinion about Stephen's mental health by either DWP or Atos.

Osborne is so concerned he writes a prevention of future deaths report. The short report (just two pages) is sent to work and pensions secretary Yvette Cooper on 30 March 2010. He writes:

> During the course of the evidence [I heard] that the trigger that [led] to his decision to take his own life was the rejection of his appeal that he was not fit for work. Mr Carre had been suffering from depression and mental illness and was receiving treatment from his general practitioner and psychiatrist for some considerable time. I feel the decision by the Department not to seek medical advice from the Claimant's own GP or psychiatrist if they are suffering a mental illness should be reviewed. Both doctors who gave evidence before me confirmed that if they had been approached they would have been willing to provide a report of Mr Carre's present condition and prognosis …

Stephen's father, Peter, has no doubt that if this advice had been sought, the outcome of his claim would have been different and 'he would in all probability still be with us today'.

It wasn't until I phoned Sarah years later that she learned of the link between Stephen's death and the WCA. She was horrified, and every detail she later learned about the WCA intensified that gnawing feeling of horror at what had happened to her beloved brother.

The prevention of future deaths report arrives at DWP's offices just days before a general election is called. It is one of many papers awaiting the attention of the incoming work and pensions secretary, Iain Duncan Smith, who is appointed after the formation of the new Conservative-Liberal Democrat coalition.

Instead of acting on the safety issues raised in the letter, Duncan Smith sticks with plans to apply the WCA to 1.6 million long-term incapacity benefit claimants, many of whom have significant and long-term mental distress.

Duncan Smith and his employment minister Chris Grayling fail to show the letter to Professor Malcolm Harrington, the independent expert they appoint to carry out the first of a series of annual reviews of the WCA. Even without seeing the letter, Harrington advises Grayling not to press ahead with the rollout of the reassessment to incapacity benefit claimants. Grayling ignores his advice.

The report Harrington issues later in the year[7] concludes that the WCA is 'impersonal' but not 'broken', although there is much to be done to make it 'fairer and more effective'.

Yvette Cooper insists years later that if she had remained as work and pensions secretary, she would have called for an immediate review of Stephen Carré's case and the process for claimants with mental distress. 'When a coroner makes a serious assessment like this, it needs to be acted upon as swiftly as possible,' she tells me.

> Ministers should have done a proper review of this and responded to the coroner's report before any decision on the roll out. We established before the 2010 election that there would need to be an independent review of the WCA and Malcolm Harrington should have been shown the coroner's report so he could consider it properly as part of the review.

It is impossible to know what a Labour government would have done. Labour's 2010 manifesto[8] promised that 'more people with disabilities and health conditions will be helped to move into work from Incapacity Benefit and Employment Support Allowance, as we extend the use of our tough-but-fair work capability test'. Matching the tough Tory talk on welfare reform, Labour claimed: 'We will reassess the Incapacity Benefit claims of 1.5 million people by 2014, as we move those able to work back into jobs.'

We also have Cooper's words in June 2010,[9] when she responds to rumoured policy changes by the new coalition. 'Labour's reforms were due to get around a million people off sickness benefits and save around £1.5 billion from introducing a new medical test and reassessing current claimants,' she says. 'That test was worked on with doctors and disability groups, and was finding more people fit for work based on proper medical evidence. We have been urging the new government to complete the implementation of those reforms and hope they will do so.'

Maybe Cooper would have seen the Stephen Carré coroner's report and realised action had to be taken. But perhaps the political pressure to follow through on its manifesto pledge – and the years of anti-claimant rhetoric – would have proved too intense, and the report would have been quietly ignored.

* * *

The question of when and how further medical evidence should be sought during the assessment process had been on the department's radar since 1992, when Mansel Aylward and his colleagues had been drawing up their 'scheme for the future control of invalidity benefit'.

But seeking this kind of evidence from consultants and GPs was time-consuming and expensive, and made it more likely that claimants would be found not fit for work. At first, Sir Leigh Lewis, DWP's permanent secretary and its most senior civil servant, asks for more information so DWP can 'complete our investigation and review our existing procedures, as you have asked, to determine the need for any changes to our current medical evidence gathering process'.

Tom Osborne tells him DWP does not need to investigate the circumstances surrounding Stephen Carré's death. That investigation has already taken place at the inquest. What DWP needs to do is look at the 'use of medical evidence'. He sends Sir Leigh a transcript of the inquest evidence.

Meanwhile, disabled activists hear of the first high-profile death to be linked to the introduction of ESA and the WCA. The little-known but highly regarded Scottish poet Paul Reekie takes his own life in June 2010. He leaves no suicide note but lays out two letters from DWP that notified him that his housing benefit and incapacity benefit were being stopped.

It is still unclear today why his incapacity benefit was stopped when the main reassessment process was not due to begin until 2011, but his death is the first to spark significant public concern about the WCA, and it leads to the formation of Black Triangle, a Scottish-based grassroots campaign of disabled activists. Black Triangle hopes to 'galvanise opposition to the current vicious attack on the fundamental human rights of disabled people' by the UK government and Atos through the WCA. Its website is dedicated to Paul Reekie's memory.

In the summer and autumn of 2010, two other new grassroots groups of disabled activists are formed. First comes the Mental Health Resistance Network, set up 'by people who live with mental distress in order to defend ourselves from the assault on us by a cruel government'. Its members are those waiting to be 'migrated' from incapacity benefit onto the new ESA, or onto jobseeker's allowance if found fit for work.

Part of that assault is the announcement from George Osborne, the new chancellor, of plans to cut spending on disability living allowance (DLA), a disability benefit that contributes towards disabled people's extra costs. Iain Duncan Smith tells MPs, in familiar DWP language, that spending on DLA has 'spiralled out of control, and the system has been vulnerable to error, abuse and, in some cases, outright fraud'.

In October, another grassroots mental health group, Mad Pride – closely linked to the Mental Health Resistance Network – takes over Hyde Park Corner to burn a two-faced effigy of David Cameron and George Osborne and protest the coalition's 'savage' welfare cuts.[10] One activist tells me during the protest that government plans to force mental health service users into work and cut their benefits are like 'throwing a hand grenade into people's lives'.

On 3 October, a third grassroots group is launched. Disabled People Against Cuts (DPAC) is formed by disabled people who march against government cuts at the beginning of the Conservative Party conference in Birmingham, many wearing 'Cuts Kill' tee-shirts. Several talk of their fears that austerity cuts will lead disabled people to take their own lives in despair. 'It's not easy now, but it's going to be even tougher,' says co-founder Eleanor Lisney. The Mental Health Resistance Network, Black Triangle, and DPAC will play critical roles in fighting the cuts to disabled people's support.

The rhetoric inside the 2010 Tory conference provides no reassurance to those protesting outside. The prime minister, David Cameron, tells Conservative members, revelling in power following their election victory in May that ended 13 years of New Labour government: 'If you really cannot work, we will always look after you. But if you can work, and refuse to work, we will not let you live off the hard work of others.'

A few weeks later, Duncan Smith tells *The Sun*[11] its readers are 'right to be angry' when they see neighbours who do not work, and that Britain used to be 'the workshop of the world' but had now 'managed to create a block of people' who

> do not add anything to the greatness of this country … They have become conditioned to be users of services, not providers of money. This is a huge part of the reason we have this massive deficit … We don't want to talk about scroungers in the future, we want to talk about British people being renowned the world over for working hard.

He says he is 'appalled' at how easy it has been in the past for people to claim incapacity benefit (IB) and defraud the system, and he suggests a large proportion are cheats. He is drawing a clear link between IB claimants and the government's budget deficit.

A DWP spokesperson later confirms to me that Duncan Smith – with his vicious scapegoating of disabled people – has been quoted accurately.

Tom Osborne's letter is all but ignored. DWP has a legal duty to respond but fails to do so. A draft response is, apparently, prepared, but it is never sent to the coroner.

Minor changes are made to the WCA, with alterations to what DWP calls 'filework guidance' introduced in December 2010,[12] informing Atos staff that if a claimant has shown 'evidence of a previous suicide attempt, suicidal ideation or self harm' in their ESA50 capability for work questionnaire, they 'must' request further medical evidence. It is far from enough, particularly because many claimants with mental distress are unable to provide such evidence.

Meanwhile, DWP has failed to tell the benefits appeal tribunal that Stephen has died, despite Peter having informed the department on 25 January. The appeal goes ahead on 20 July. When the tribunal staff call out Stephen's name, Peter says: 'Yes, here.' And he holds up his son's ashes.

The tribunal casts doubt upon the validity of the assessment, not least because the Atos report was written eight days after the test was carried out and referred to the claimant as 'Paul David Carter'. The case is referred upwards to a district tribunal judge.

The second tribunal takes place in August 2011, and concludes that the assessment report is a 'suspect document', and that Stephen should have scored enough points to be found not fit for work. DWP eventually reverses its original decision and agrees Stephen was incapable of returning to work. Peter forwards the back-payments to the solicitor acting for Stephen's children. Many, many more such transactions will take place over the next decade.

PART III

2010–14
The Coalition, Austerity, and Deaths by Welfare

11

Atos, Activism, and the Climate of Panic

For the first few years of the coalition, it is disabled activists who spend their time and resources raising concerns about the harm DWP is causing. The media report the occasional death, but the research is carried out at grassroots level, because it is disabled people who are experiencing the brutal impact of welfare reform. In September 2011, the Mental Health Resistance Network submits evidence to Professor Harrington's second review of the work capability assessment (WCA).[1] The network describes its members' 'deep distress at the manner in which these changes have been taking place', and their 'relapses, including episodes of self harm and suicide attempts, together with requiring increases in medication and even hospitalisation in anticipation of their reassessment'. They say the incapacity benefit reassessment process 'is happening at a time when mental health services are being cut'. There is 'a climate of panic' but little support available. They stress the significant problems faced by many members in self-reporting how their mental distress affects them, while it is particularly difficult to relay this impact in a face-to-face assessment to 'someone who is a stranger and with whom one has had no opportunity to build trust or who has limited time'.

They tell Harrington:

> We therefore emphasize the importance of evidence from our health care professionals. Importantly, we think that the DWP should take responsibility for obtaining this evidence, that it should not be left to the vagaries of our available support and our own condition to ensure that all evidence is made available to the decision maker.

This criticism has sat right at the heart of concerns about the department's assessment processes since the early 1990s, when Aylward and his colleagues set out to sideline the medical professionals who knew claimants best and transfer power to DWP and their specialist assessors.

Labour – now led by Ed Miliband – continues to provide political cover for the coalition's welfare reforms. In his 2011 party conference speech,[2] shadow work and pensions secretary Liam Byrne says: 'Let's face the tough truth – that many people on the doorstep at the last election felt that too often we were for shirkers, not workers.' The media are still mirroring this rhetoric. A report commissioned by the disabled people's organisation Inclusion London[3] shows the proportion of news stories about disability benefit fraud more than doubled between 2004–05 and 2010–11. When focus groups described a typical news story about disability, they usually mentioned benefit fraud and suggested as many as 70 per cent of claims were fraudulent, referring to articles they had read. In fact, government figures show incapacity benefit fraud at just £20 million a year, or 0.3 per cent of spending.

Meanwhile, the insurance industry's links with the government are as close as ever. Unum launches a major campaign, aimed at persuading workers to ask their employers to provide income protection insurance (IPI), which will pay out if they become disabled or ill and cannot work. The campaign begins just as the government launches its programme to reassess 1.5 million claimants of incapacity benefit through the work capability assessment.

Unum sponsors fringe meetings at the three main party conferences in 2011. When asked after the Conservative fringe if his company had influenced the welfare reform agenda, Unum's chief executive, Jack McGarry, tells me: 'We haven't tried to influence the welfare agenda around reducing welfare or making it harder to claim. To my knowledge we have not done that.'

Tim Jackson, Unum's head of marketing strategy, says the publicity around the tougher benefits regime is particularly raising awareness among those in the 'squeezed middle' income bracket. 'What welfare reform does really is highlight the problem to them,' he says, 'so now is a good time to talk about it. The state provides a great safety net for those who are most at risk and exposed, but for those in the squeezed middle range it will not support their lifestyles.' He denies that Unum's marketing push was timed to coincide with the launch of the government's reassessment programme. 'There was no connection with that whatsoever,' he insists. Apparently, the timing was just a coincidence.

One disabled campaigner highlighting Unum's influence is retired healthcare professional and Women's Royal Air Force veteran Mo Stewart (a pseudonym). Stewart first became interested in the private sector's role in welfare reform after being visited by an Atos doctor, who was conducting a medical assessment for her war pension.

She tells me: 'The doctor who visited me actually refused to offer any form of ID, resisted eye contact, advised I was only "permitted" to speak in answer to any questions and produced a totally bogus report.' Stewart will spend much of the next decade researching links between companies such as Unum and the destruction of the welfare state.

Another disabled activist concerned about Unum is Debbie Jolly. A DPAC co-founder, she will play a hugely significant – but largely unrecognised – role in bridging the gap between the disabled people's movement and academic research into the impact of austerity, until her death in November 2016. In 2012, she publishes an influential blog on DPAC's website,[4] warning that the number of suicides 'brought about by the fear and misery imposed on disabled people through the current neoliberal regime is likely to grow'. This, she says, 'is about denying benefits, denying illness and denying disability: It's about something Unum have a successful history of: denying pay outs for disabled people while capitalising on fear and risk.'

The Welfare Reform Act[5] receives royal assent in March 2012. The legislation introduces universal credit, the bedroom tax, and personal independence payment, the new disability benefit that will replace working-age disability living allowance and which ministers hope will cut spending in that area by 20 per cent. There is also a new twelve-month limit for those receiving the contributory form of ESA who are placed in the work-related activity group.

In July 2012, the high court grants permission for a judicial review case backed by the Mental Health Resistance Network. With the help of solicitors from Public Law Project, they highlight how the WCA discriminates against autistic people, people with mental distress and those with learning difficulties. They want to ensure that DWP and Atos have all the medical evidence they need to decide an ESA claim fairly. But DWP fails to tell the network's legal team about the Stephen Carré prevention of future deaths report or other secret documents whose existence will only emerge in later years.

The following month, disabled activists from DPAC – working with UK Uncut – target Atos in the run-up to the London 2012 Paralympic Games, underscoring the hypocrisy of Atos sponsoring London 2012.

They launch the Anti Atos Games with their own opening ceremony, parodying the WCA. They also deliver a coffin full of messages to Atos's headquarters in central London, aiming to draw attention to the estimated 1,100 people who died within six months of being found fit for work, over just an eight-month period. Hundreds of activists attend the protest. Two documentaries exposing the flaws in the WCA are broadcast in the same week. DPAC activist and author Ellen Clifford will write later that, by the end of the week, Atos 'had become a household name'.[6]

In September, Labour MP Michael Meacher raises the case of Colin Traynor in the Commons.[7] Traynor had received incapacity benefit because of his lifelong epilepsy. He was deemed 'unemployable' by a government disability employment contractor. Three years later, he was told to attend a work capability assessment. He failed to provide any further medical evidence and was found fit for work.

'This caused Colin a lot of stress and anxiety,' Meacher tells fellow MPs. 'He was worried about losing his home, not being able to pay his bills and even worried about not being able to afford good food to eat. He was informed that the decision would have to go to an appeal and could take as long as nine months.'

From December 2011 to April 2012, his health deteriorated, his seizures increased due to the stress, and he lost weight. Following evidence from his GP and an epilepsy specialist nurse, DWP changed the original decision and placed him in the ESA work-related activity group, for those 'expected to undertake activity to support their return to the labour market'. On 3 April 2012, the stress and anxiety led to a massive seizure. He died at home on his own, aged 29. In a letter to Meacher, Colin's family said they held the government, David Cameron and Iain Duncan Smith 'personally responsible' for his death.

DWP minister Mark Hoban tells MPs the reassessment programme 'is a key part of our reform agenda' and that a review found the department 'correctly applied the procedures for incapacity benefit reassessment in this case'. He blames Colin Traynor for not providing the necessary medical evidence after he was found fit for work.

In October 2012, George Osborne delivers what will become a notorious speech to the Conservative Party conference in Birmingham.[8] It is wrong, Osborne tells party members, for someone to be better off on benefits than they would be in work. This is why he insisted on a benefit cap, so 'no family can earn more out of work than the average family earns in work'.

> Where is the fairness, we ask, for the shift-worker, leaving home in the dark hours of the early morning, who looks up at the closed blinds of their next door neighbour sleeping off a life on benefits? When we say we're all in this together, we speak for that worker … We modern Conservatives represent all those who aspire, all who work, save and hope, all who feel a responsibility to put in, not just take out.

Osborne's speech will further incite the abuse and harassment of disabled people claiming benefits. In the post-2010 years, there will be repeated warnings that the government's presentation of its reforms – and the way it briefs the media – is whipping up hostility towards disabled people, and leading to disability hate crime. It leads to misleading and offensive headlines such as 'Time's up for the shirking classes' in the *Daily Mail* and 'Sick benefits: 75 per cent are faking' in the *Express*, in July 2011[9], and the *Daily Mail*'s 'Workshy map of Britain' the following year.[10]

The following year, a disabled crossbench peer, the Countess of Mar, will tell a Liberal Democrat minister[11] that disabled people are facing public hostility, with strangers accosting them in the street and accusing them of faking their impairments. 'I don't need to remind you what happened in 1930s Germany when disabled people and older people were regarded as a burden on the state,' she says. 'We do not want to sleepwalk into that situation.'

Years later, in 2017, Theresia Degener, chair of the UN committee on the rights of persons with disabilities, will warn during an interview with the BBC – in comments that are not broadcast – that disabled people could be at risk of violence, and even 'killings and euthanasia', because of their portrayal by the UK government and media as 'parasites' who live on benefits.[12]

In November 2012, Spartacus, a network of disabled researchers, publishes its 'People's Review of the Work Capability Assessment'.[13] The report details cases involving ESA claimants who have killed themselves or otherwise died after being found fit for work. Many describe their experiences at the hands of Atos assessors. A woman who accompanied her husband to his WCA says: 'I can honestly say there are lies that go into that assessment. I do shorthand and I took down word for word my husband's whole assessment. What actually came back was practically the opposite of everything he said.'

Four days later, Dr Bill Gunnyeon, successor to Mansel Aylward as DWP's chief medical adviser, who has overall responsibility for WCA policy, provides his first written statement to the Mental Health Resistance Network court case. He suggests that asking GPs to provide further medical evidence for all ESA applicants with mental health conditions would be burdensome. Atos can issue requests to GPs 'where relevant and appropriate' and it would be 'unreasonable to increase this burden without evidence to demonstrate that a blanket requirement would significantly aid the process by providing relevant additional material'.

The following day, Professor Harrington publishes his third review of the WCA.[14] He still believes the assessment should not be scrapped, but – even though he has not been shown the Stephen Carré coroner's report – he says: 'Decision-makers should actively consider the need to seek further documentary evidence in every claimant's case. The final decision should be justified where this is not sought.' The claimants in the Mental Health Resistance Network court case adopt this recommendation as the 'reasonable adjustment' they want DWP to make under the Equality Act. The department starts work on a pilot.

* * *

17 January 2013. Michael Meacher secures another Commons debate.[15] He has been sent nearly 300 case histories of people affected by the WCA. He tells fellow MPs: 'I cannot begin to do justice to the feelings of distress, indignation, fear, helplessness and indeed widespread anger at the way they have been treated.'

He raises concerns about Atos's chief medical officer, Professor Michael O'Donnell, who has joined the company from Unum, which was described in 2005 as an 'outlaw company' by a US official, partly because it is regarded as a 'disability denial factory'.

His Labour colleague Kevan Jones says the government has 'blood on its hands' from the deaths of disabled people caused by the WCA. Jones says DWP has been asked to record the number of cases of suicide connected with the WCA but has refused.

John McDonnell, later to be shadow chancellor under Jeremy Corbyn, says the system is unreformable and 'we will be to blame for every injury, every harm, every suicide, every death as a result of the system if we do not do something now to scrap it'.

But DWP minister Mark Hoban holds the department line. He speaks of 'the myth that the WCA is not fit for purpose'. 'The assessment we inherited needed refinement,' he says.

> That is why we accepted and have largely implemented more than 40 of [Harrington's] recommendations over the past two years. That is why twice as many people have gone into the support group in comparison with when ESA was introduced ... demonis-

ing the work capability assessment does not help our constituents and does not address their concerns.

In April, DWP begins its lengthy rollout of personal independence payment (PIP), the new disability benefit that is replacing working-age disability living allowance. The PIP assessment process will soon be drawing much of the same criticism as the dysfunctional WCA.

As the new benefit is launched – with the intention of cutting spending and the number of claimants by a fifth – David Cameron authors an article in *The Sun*[16] in which he says the welfare system 'has become a lifestyle choice for some' which is 'causing resentment'. Much of that resentment has been whipped up by politicians like Cameron, George Osborne, and Iain Duncan Smith, and the previous Labour government.

He tells *Sun* readers: 'We are working our way through everyone on what was called "Incapacity Benefit", more often known as "the sick", to see who can actually work, particularly if they are given some help … This is a Government for hard-working people – and that's the way it will stay.'

The first of a series of whistleblowers from DWP and its contractors comes forward to describe what it is like working for Atos. Dr Greg Wood has quit his job as an Atos assessor after he is asked yet again to change a WCA report. Speaking to the BBC,[17] he says he believes the assessments are 'unfair' and 'skewed against the claimant'. He describes a WCA training session and being given guidance that made it much easier for claimants to be found fit for work. He is told that if a claimant can press a button, they should get no points for manual dexterity, and if they can wash and dress themselves, 'they have enough drive and concentration to do a job'. He eventually quits when told by two managers to reduce the number of points awarded to a claimant with significant mental distress, who he knew had chronic psychosis.

The upper tribunal delivers its judgment on the Mental Health Resistance Network case, concluding that DWP breached its duty to make reasonable adjustments under the Equality Act by leaving claimants to collect their own medical evidence.[18] It finds DWP's policies put people with mental health conditions and learning difficulties and autistic people at a substantial disadvantage, because many of them have problems filling in forms and seeking additional evidence. It orders DWP to investigate how to ensure the necessary medical evidence can be obtained. DWP tells the tribunal the judgment goes substantially further than the pilot it had proposed. It suggests a new pilot, while also appealing the judgment.

This means further delays to attempts to make the system safer. As Dr China Mills says later,[19] DWP is using delay as a strategy to avoid accountability and deny justice, which will lead to the further build-up of 'incremental harms'. DWP, she says, is weaponising time.

12
The Death of David Clapson

March 2022. There are clusters of trees across the park. In a corner is a fenced-in playground. A storm has left branches scattered across the heavy ground. In the centre of Bedwell Shops Park is an oak sapling, two wooden supports holding it almost upright. At the foot of the sapling is a bronze plaque, laid into stone that is speckled grey, black and white. On the plaque are the words:

David George Clapson
As we watch this mighty Oak grow
the memory of a gentle man lives in our
hearts forever
Loved by all who knew him
24245667 L/Cpl CLAPSON DG

At the edge of the park, looking out across the trees, the sapling, and the plaque, are two blocks of three-storey flats, each a mix of beige brickwork and white vinyl doors and windows. Number 21 of the right-hand block, Hillside House, was David Clapson's flat.

July 2013. The country, and Stevenage, are in the middle of a heatwave, temperatures reaching into the high 20s. David Clapson's unclothed body is sprawled across the hallway of 21 Hillside House. A few feet from his body is a pile of CVs. David has written: 'I am a multi-skilled, hardworking and efficient individual with extensive warehouse experience and a proven track record of ensuring the smooth functioning and running of all warehouse activities …' There is just 5p credit on David's mobile phone, and £3.44 in his bank account.

* * *

They were a close family. David, his sister Gill, younger by three years, and their parents. They lived in Essex Road, Islington, in north London, until David was ten, before moving to Stevenage. Their mum would live in the same house in West Close for the next 47 years.

Gill remembers their annual late-July beach holidays, digging holes in the sand together. How the children from West Close used to visit the local community centre for Saturday morning pictures, on the edge of Bedwell Shops Park. In later years, David would take his mum to the centre for lunch after she developed dementia. He and his friends would play football in what they called The Dip, a sunken patch of greenery near West Close. 'We were very close when we were younger,' says Gill. 'He was a good brother, and we used to do a lot together. I got stuck up a tree, and he came and got me down. Some brothers would have left you there, wouldn't they ...'

David was a quiet person, his sister told me; he bonded with people of all ages, but he also liked to spend time on his own. He loves music, particularly rock and metal bands such as Black Sabbath, Deep Purple and Led Zeppelin, and punk bands like Radical Dance Faction and Stevenage's Scum of Toytown. He visits Germany with a friend for the beer festival, and is into motorcycle racing, speedway, cricket. He enjoys history documentaries, and loves to read. He was, says Gill, 'a quiet, private, proud man who didn't like to ask for help'.

David joins the Royal Signals, the shortest member of the regiment. He serves for five years, three years in Germany and two in Northern Ireland as a combat radio operator, at the height of The Troubles in the 1970s. When he comes home on leave, David meets up with his sister and they go clubbing with his friend.

He returns to Stevenage when he leaves the army, returning with his new wife, a strong-willed young woman from Belfast, and a golden labrador. They marry in around 1976 and the marriage lasts until 1988.

After leaving the army, David works for 16 years with BT, before working as a delivery driver and spells as a warehouse operative with Allied Bakeries and Dixon's. But he struggles when he leaves BT and their 'tower of strength' mother becomes ill with dementia. He needed his mother and his wife to help him run his life, says Gill. After his divorce, he loses his home following a struggle with his finances, moves in with his mother and becomes her carer. He struggles with forms and paying bills. 'David didn't open envelopes,' says Gill.

David spends seven years looking after his mother. 'We probably kept her at home longer than we should have done because I was worried about what would happen to David,' says Gill. When she moves into a care home in 2010, David finds a place at The Haven, a hostel in Stevenage. Gill takes him to Citizens Advice, and they help him claim jobseeker's allowance (JSA). The Haven finds him a flat overlooking the park where he and Gill played together as children.

His cousin, Irene Usher, lives just 100 yards away from David's new flat, and remembers him visiting to watch televised Arsenal games. 'He was such a lovely, cheerful bloke. He never looked on the downside.' She now regrets not asking him to join them for dinner, but she hadn't wanted to interfere. He never suggests he is struggling for money.

After David starts claiming JSA, he takes courses, including one on how to drive forklift trucks. He is placed on a Work Programme scheme run by the private sector contractor Seetec. He takes part in two work placements, at Poundland and B&Q, and enjoys them, and seeks further placements, but is told to 'give someone else a chance'. He asks the jobcentre for extra help, but they tell him, 'We're not here to help you get a job, that's the other place.'

He often struggles for money, and his sister will take a taxi to Hillside House and bring him a food parcel, although he never asks her for help. It is the same with his friends. He doesn't like to ask them to buy him drinks when he can't return the favour, so he often stays home.

His closest friend, Alan Knowler, remembers David as 'the most loveable bloke going, so sociable and happy'. David and Alan drink together at the Red Lion in Stevenage. David was ten years older. They would travel to Peterborough to watch the speedway, and they visit Glastonbury festival in 1986. 'All he wanted was a quiet life to do his own thing,' says Alan, when Gill and I meet him at the Red Lion one Saturday afternoon in 2022. 'But if he could help you out, he would help you out. He was right into his history, politics. He never watched mainstream TV, he would always be watching a documentary, or something about history.'

In later years, David was 'always skint,' says Alan. 'I would phone him up and ask if he wanted a beer. He would work out what he could spend. He would say, "I can get two pints this week," and he would buy me a beer.' He was well known and well liked at the pub. 'All Dave wanted was to get a job and a job that he could get enough money to buy his food for the week and pay his bills and enough money to come out and have a drink and buy a little bit of doobie [cannabis].'

Alan remembers walking back from a party and asking David why he was struggling to walk. A friend at the Red Lion tells him he had had similar symptoms and was diagnosed with diabetes. 'We kept on at him that he should get checked out for diabetes,' says Alan. Eventually, David visits his GP, and is told he has type one diabetes.

Alan remembers David having to attend work search meetings organised by Seetec twice a week. He never missed an appointment. Shortly before he died, he is told to attend a three-day computer course, where he would be 'sat in a classroom with a load of other people and be talked to'. Alan says this would never have worked. 'Dave needed someone to sit down next to him and show him the ins and outs.'

In 2010 or 2011, David's JSA is stopped because he fails to fill in a form correctly. He runs out of money, has no food and is taking insulin to try to control his diabetes. His neighbours hear a noise and find him collapsed on the floor. The paramedics say he had been 'an hour from dying'. He spends several days in hospital and is told never to take his insulin without food. Gill asks the jobcentre how this could have happened, but 'no-one seemed concerned'. DWP would later be unable to find any record of her call. David persuades her not to complain, telling her: 'Sis, don't cause a scene, I'll sort it out.'

On 3 July 2013, David is sent a letter by DWP, telling him a 'doubt has arisen on your entitlement to Jobseeker's Allowance' because he missed a Work Programme appointment. A second letter, twelve days later, tells him he is being sanctioned for a month, from 12 July until 8 August. He is told his payments of £71.70 a week will resume from 9 August. Both letters are later found unopened. 'David just didn't open letters,' said Gill. 'That was it. His money was stopped.' No attempt is made to check whether removing his only source of income could have a drastic impact on his health.

David does not find out until he tries to withdraw money from the cashpoint. On 16 July, he visits the jobcentre, and may have been told he can apply for a hardship loan. It is unclear exactly what is said during the conversation, and why he doesn't apply, but the form is eleven pages long and David struggles with paperwork. Claimants can apply immediately if staff decide that, because of a health condition, the sanction will cause a greater deterioration than in a normal healthy adult. 'They say they followed procedures, and no errors were made,' says Gill. 'David was an insulin-dependent diabetic. By stopping his money, they took away his lifeline.' He isn't due to receive any money again until 8 August.

David tells Alan he has been sanctioned. 'If they had told him about an appointment down the dole, he wouldn't have missed it,' Alan tells me years later. 'It was the fact that they had sent him it in a letter and he hadn't opened the letter.' David asks his friend how he is going to put money on his electricity key. 'I have got bills due,' he says. Alan asks him what he will do. 'I have no idea,' he says. 'I need to sit down and think about it. I'll be in touch.'

David has been struggling since their mother died. 'He was depressed because he was very close to our mum,' says Gill. 'She was our tower of strength. I don't think she worried about me so much, but you could see when she used to look at her Davey, I think she worried about him.' He has collapsed several times and been taken to hospital in the ten years since his diabetes diagnosis, the last time shortly before he died. 'The DWP knew he was an insulin-dependent diabetic. The last few times I saw him he looked like an old man. He just looked old and he looked tired, he was dishevelled. He was just struggling, he was really struggling.'

She is finding it increasingly difficult to get hold of David on his pay-as-you-go mobile. She suspects he ran out of credit. But on the Thursday afternoon (18 July), he answers the phone. 'We had the best conversation ever,' said Gill. 'He said he'd applied for a job at Lidl and was waiting to hear. He was quite chirpy, not a word about anything.'

Alan is becoming worried at not hearing from David and begins phoning their friends. Early afternoon on Saturday, he calls Gill. He says they are worried and tells her David has been sanctioned. 'I didn't even know what sanctions were,' said Gill. 'I'd never heard of them. I was living in London, so Alan said, "Don't worry, we're going to go round to see if he's OK."'

Alan is working as a painter and decorator, so he puts a ladder on his roof-rack and drives to David's flat with two of their friends. He takes the ladder and puts it against the wall of David's flat, near the kitchen and living-room windows, but cannot see anything to worry about. In the meantime, one of his friends finds the front door is unlocked. 'I heard my mate shout that he was in the hallway, and he didn't look good.'

David is lying on his back, naked, with his head near the kitchen door and his feet near the living-room door. They check his pulse. He is dead. There is no electricity in the flat. The fridge is empty. A neighbour will later say they heard beeping from the flat. Gill thinks that was because the electricity had run out. Near David's body is a pile of CVs.

There is no food in the flat except six tea-bags, two tins of tomato soup and a tin of pilchards, as well as four beer cans, an empty bottle of wine, and a small amount of cannabis resin. An oven tray, containing some cooked sausage and chips, has been left in the kitchen. His electricity key ran out at some point before his body was found. He needed electricity to keep his insulin chilled in the fridge. It's not clear when it ran out.

For Gill, one of the most painful pieces of information to emerge after her brother's death was that a letter from BT, containing a cheque for £750, was one of the unopened pieces of correspondence found scattered about the flat.

Gill is still tormented by not knowing when her brother died. Was it Thursday or Friday? She struggled afterwards thinking about these two days, that she was going about her life, unaware that at some point – she will never know when – her brother had collapsed and died, alone in his flat.

* * *

The crematorium is packed, with some people having to stand outside, including some of David's biker mates. The wake is at the Red Lion.

The post-mortem concludes that David's stomach was empty at the time of his death. The cause of death was fatal diabetic keto-acidosis.

Office of the District Manager, St Albans Jobcentre
29 May 2014

Dear Mrs Thompson

Please accept my apology for the delay in replying to you. As promised, I have looked at the records we have concerning our interaction with Mr Clapson during the time he was receiving benefit. Your brother did inform us of his diabetes and that he was insulin dependent. However, he assured us that this was controlled. I have not found any errors made on his claim or with the course of action we took with him in relation to his Jobseeker's Allowance.

I could not find a record of the telephone call you made to us of Mr Clapson's collapse for which I do apologise. A record should have been made of this on his case … From our telephone conversation I fully understand that your brother was a private person who did not like to ask for help. We had referred him to our work provider Seetec who specialise in helping our more vulnerable claimants. This meant that he was not visiting the Jobcentre regularly. However, we and our work providers do rely on people to tell us that they are having difficulties with what we ask them to do, so that we can review the situation.

With all our decisions which affect payments of benefit the claimant has the right to ask us to reconsider our decision and has an opportunity to give us their reasons as to why they failed to comply with us. Claimants who do have their benefit suspended are able to apply for hardship payments.

There is no inquest. The coroner decides David found it difficult to control his diabetes, and because of the sausage and chips, although his stomach was empty, he had food available and chose not to eat it. He attributes his death to natural causes, and says the benefit sanction that left him destitute had not helped cause his death. David died on 20 July and had just £3.44 to last him until 8 August.

It takes a couple of months for Gill to begin to ask questions. She had been comforted by there being no signs that David died in pain. But then she is told he had no food in his stomach, and she makes the link with the sanction. Gill is not a natural campaigner, but she is the only one left to fight for David. She has no other siblings; both their parents are dead. 'I felt I had to do it,' she tells me later. 'I don't know what my mum and dad would have said because they were very, very quiet, very private. We were a family that didn't do confrontation. We didn't argue, we didn't fight. We were just a very quiet and private family that used to go for walks.'

But she wants justice for her brother. 'David could have died any time with his diabetes, but that doesn't make it right. Sanctions aren't necessary. All they do is impose misery on people.' So she decides to fight. She starts to hear of other deaths, and speaks to her local newspaper and then national newspapers like the *Mirror* and *The Guardian*. She starts a petition for an inquiry into the sanctions regime.

She opens the envelopes from David's flat and finds the two appointments he missed. Then she researches other victims of the sanctions regime. 'I want to know how the Department of Work and Pensions can justify welfare sanctions that are driving people to foodbanks and leading to starvation and death,' she writes on the Change.org petition web page. An oak tree is planted in David's memory, in Bedwell Shops Park. Gill and her husband Michael attend the unveiling.

More than 200,000 people sign Gill's petition, and she speaks at a *Daily Mirror* fringe event at the Labour conference in September 2014. The following month, the work and pensions committee – chaired by disabled Labour MP Anne Begg – announces an inquiry into benefit sanctions policy.

DWP figures show the number of ESA claimants (those in the work-related activity group) being sanctioned increased by nearly 580 per cent between March 2013 and March 2014. Gill tells the committee in written evidence: 'There used to be a time if you missed your job centre meeting and had a long term illness like diabetes or was vulnerable there would be concern and outreach by job centre staff. Now they cut off your benefits.'

In November, Gill joins Cathie Wood, sister of another DWP victim, and speaks about David's death at a public meeting in David Cameron's Witney constituency, organised by the Green Party.

The following February, Esther McVey, the employment minister, gives evidence to the committee. 'There are categorically no targets; there is no harassment,' she tells Labour's Debbie Abrahams.[1] She insists the government is 'supporting the most vulnerable' and that sanctions help people into work. 'We know it works,' she says. David's case is not mentioned, but Gill and Michael have been sitting behind McVey and listening to her angrily defend the sanctions regime. As McVey prepares to leave, Gill places a picture of her brother in his army uniform on the desk in front of the minister. 'My brother is dead, and he wasn't a criminal,' Gill says. 'You took away his lifeline.'

'It's a complex case, I'm sorry,' McVey replies.

'There's nothing complex about it,' Gill says. 'He was a diabetic and starving. A diabetic cannot wait two weeks.' Michael picks up David's picture, which McVey has left on the desk.

David Cameron is asked about David's case and his wider austerity cuts on *The Andrew Marr Show*,[2] a few weeks before the 2015 general election. Cameron says 'councils have hardship funds for exactly those sorts of tragic cases' but adds:

> People watching this programme who pay their taxes, who work very hard, they don't pay their taxes so people can sign on and show no effort at getting a job. As I put it on the steps of Downing Street, those who can, should; those who can't, we always help. That is the principle that should always underline a compassionate benefits system.

Gill tries to confront Iain Duncan Smith at a constituency hustings, accompanied by the *Mirror*'s Ros Wynne Jones. He doesn't turn up. He is re-elected and continues as work and pensions secretary.

In October, Gill gives written evidence to the UN committee on the rights of persons with disabilities, which is investigating allegations of 'systematic and grave' violations of disabled people's human rights, focused on DWP policies. She writes: 'David missed one or two appointments and for that he was sanctioned and died. If he had been a criminal he would have had a trial, with judge, jury, and a proper defence.'

The following year, backed by a crowd-funding appeal,[3] Gill asks the coroner to reconsider his refusal to hold an inquest. She is represented by solicitors Leigh Day, who will take on several other high-profile DWP cases.

The coroner refuses to open an inquest and says David 'made a lifestyle choice about how to deploy his limited funds', that he was 'extremely poor at controlling his diabetes', had 'ready access to food when he died', and 'chose' not to open his correspondence. He says he had 'access to a small amount of money'. This was the £3.44 in his bank account, not enough to draw out of a cashpoint machine. Gill says she was distraught when she read this portrayal of her brother.

Leigh Day, through Gill's solicitor Merry Varney, seeks a judicial review. Barristers Caoilfhionn Gallagher and Jesse Nicholls argue that 'when enforcing benefit sanctions on those dependent on welfare benefits, the State is under a duty to put in place systems, precautions and guidance that will protect the right to life of those affected by the benefit sanctions regime and guard against the risks posed by such a regime'.

But the high court refuses Gill permission to continue with her claim, with the judge accepting the coroner's position. 'I felt I failed them,' Gill tells me. 'I raised all that money and it got rejected. All I wanted was for this just to stop, for this suffering to stop. That's all I've ever wanted, and I didn't get that.'

13

The Death of Mark Wood

A market researcher knocks on the front door of 16 Chetwynd Mead. It is Friday 9 August 2013. There is no answer.

The house is on the edge of the village of Bampton, in the Witney constituency of prime minister David Cameron. It is two-bedroomed, semi-detached, built from golden Cotswold stone, set slightly back from a road that winds through a cul-de-sac, just a minute's walk from the flat farmlands and oak woodlands of the Thames Vale.

It is only when the researcher pushes a business card through the brass letterbox that he notices the smell and sees the flies. He knocks on neighbours' doors. One of them says the occupant has been ill. No one has seen him for more than a week.

When the police force entry, they find the body of Mark Wood, dressed in black trousers and a black jacket. His feet are on the floor, and he is lying on his back on his bed. The bed is downstairs, on the tiled floor of the kitchen-dining-room. The room opens onto the living room, where bin-liners contain papers, clothes, and other items.

Mark had last been seen by a neighbour eleven days earlier. His body weighs just five-and-a-half stone.

> Even before I got MCS [multiple chemical sensitivity*] I found it very difficult to manage my life, because of my personality, mental health and 'autistic' difficulties and needed a lot of support from the Twelve Step Fellowship, the mental health services and periodically my family, in order to keep going and living independently.

* Multiple chemical sensitivity: a condition triggered by exposure to low levels of chemicals.

I was always under stress and having crises – emotional, financial, relationships, practical etc.

During one period of extreme distress [winter 1995/6] I had three months of inpatient psychiatric treatment and the diagnoses I was given made sense of the difficulties I had in coping with life: Addictive personality (in active recovery from addictions to alcohol, drugs, sex, cigarettes); Obsessive compulsive disorder; Anxiety and phobias; Depression; Some autistic problems (possibly due to minimal brain damage) which makes it difficult for me to organise day-to-day life and to relate to other people.

However, MCS has made my situation much worse … Most days I get an exposure of some kind, which makes me feel ill and exhausted and prevents me carrying out any plan I may have had. This makes me emotionally very stressed and increases my long-standing depression …

My anxious and obsessive nature seems to get me trapped in endless worrying. I am easily distracted by anxieties. I also find life too complicated and often find it difficult to make decisions about what to do. My phobic tendencies also restrict what I can do. For example I have developed phobias to certain places and can no longer go there because they induce major panic attacks …

Although I am intelligent, articulate and able to have a good abstract discussion, bewilderingly I find it difficult to manage day to day practicalities and affairs, to manage complex information and to make balanced decisions. I cannot keep to a routine, however hard I try …

Relationships are difficult for me as well because of my autistic traits … All in all I feel very fragile – physically and mentally and know that I could not cope with the working environment. (Extracts from account written by Jill Gant, Mark Wood's mother, in 2004 as part of his application for incapacity benefit)

Mark's mother, Jill Gant, remembers him as a 'placid' baby. She caught German measles when she was seven months pregnant, and had flu with a high temperature the day before giving birth on 25

January 1969, in Bromley, south-east London. Otherwise, the birth was normal.

She remembers her son laughing as he played physical games with his father, and how he loved their two cats. He used to follow his older sister Cathie around but did not otherwise seem interested in things around him. As a toddler, Jill would say later, he was 'passive, introverted, excruciatingly self-conscious and very easily embarrassed and humiliated'.

Mark hated clutter, and he would occasionally gather up the toys scattered around his bedroom, put them in a bag and dump them outside the door. The exasperation of those around him at his failure to listen to instructions, to socialise, to meet his family's expectations, was met with resistance. 'I think he was engulfed by us all, particularly me, and withdrew to a safe place and fantasised,' Jill would write later. 'I was never able to achieve the emotional rapport with him as a child and as a teenager that I did with my daughter. He would never allow me to cuddle him.' He would tell his mother later that he always felt that he was not doing what was required of him, but never seemed to know what that was.

He had been closest to his father, Michael, but Michael was descending gradually into alcoholism, which would result in divorce when Mark was about twelve. Jill later married John Gant, much more happily, and he became a supportive, avuncular step-father.

Cathie remembers her brother adoring animals and nature and said he 'couldn't bear cruelty to any living thing', and was 'super sensitive', which often left him overwhelmed. His life at primary school was mostly marred by criticism and humiliation, and a lack of patience and encouragement from teachers.

These problems continued into secondary school – his parents had sent him to an independent day school – where his lack of lateral thinking became more apparent. He once told his mother: 'Teachers keep saying to me, "Just use your common sense." What is common sense? I don't seem to have it.'

Although it didn't show in his academic results, Mark was a talented artist and musician. He found it difficult to read music, but taught himself electric guitar, and played and improvised beautifully. He became interested in becoming famous through joining a band. But his social anxieties remained, and grew. He was 'acutely aware of being looked at', says his mother, which often prevented him leaving the house without a friend by his side.

After passing six O-levels, he stayed on at school, but it was, his mother says, 'a disaster'. She had to force him out of bed every morning, and he was disruptive in class. He left at the end of the first year of sixth form, so the school found him an administrative job with Bromley council. It lasted nine months. He was told he was failing to take on routine instructions, and that his attitude towards work was 'totally unenthusiastic'. This would be his last permanent job.

Jill says the job highlighted some of the lifelong challenges Mark would face. He had an 'inability to hold practical information'. He was so shy he would never ask his manager for more work because he knew everyone would be looking at him. 'He was absolutely paralysed by this problem of not wanting people to look at him.'

Jill and her new husband were moving to Derbyshire, where she had secured a new job, but Mark did not want to join them. Instead, they found him a housing association flat in Penge. He lived there for eleven years but his life was, in his mother's words, 'chaotic and punctuated with crises'. He became an alcoholic and then, with the help of Alcoholics Anonymous, entered recovery.

In 1995, harassment by a neighbour forces him from the flat in Penge. He moves to a basement flat in the heart of London, a short distance from Baker Street.

The following year, a crisis leads to an emergency admission for more than two months of inpatient mental health treatment at the Churchill Clinic in south-east London, funded from his mother's pension, and then briefly as a day patient.

One of his alcohol counsellors advises him to keep away from his family, to enable him to develop independence and recover from his addiction. That idea 'became indelibly fixed in his mind', says Jill. This mindset would eventually have a tragic impact.

In 2001, his girlfriend, a young art student he had met in London, asks him to visit her in Japan. She had lived with him in his flat, but never quite understood why he had no money and could not find a job. He buys a ticket but leaves the plane before it takes off because he feels claustrophobic. He turns up at his mother's home in Derbyshire with an envelope full of debts. They pay off £2,500 and deal with another £1,500 of arrears.

After becoming increasingly depressed, he tries again to fly to Japan, but once more leaves the plane before take-off. He makes it at the third attempt, and spends a month with his girlfriend and her family.

'Mark was stoic,' says Jill. 'He was extraordinary. He would have felt that overwhelming anxiety on the third occasion just as much as the first two, but his need to go out there, his need to see this girl and to have a relationship and to do something exciting was greater than this fear, so he made it to Tokyo.' The trip does not go well. His girlfriend's parents cannot cope with his chain-smoking. The relationship – the only one he would ever have – ends after his return to England.

Mark is desperate to live an independent life. He is signing on, receiving income support, occasionally with an addition for incapacity, but no one believes he is fit for work, or ever will be. He manages a brief stay with his parents in January 2003, but they have never seen him so distressed. He speaks in tears of his daily calls to Samaritans. Eventually, after many changes of mind, his acute anxiety in their presence drives him to return to London.

The following year, the years of living in a basement flat just a few feet from a traffic-clogged street causes his health to collapse, with what is later diagnosed as multiple chemical sensitivity. 'Eventually it made him really ill, and he was under stress the whole time,' says Jill. 'He only had to have a whiff of a synthetic chemical and he was ill again, really ill.'

He leaves the flat, and begins sleeping rough, busking for money. He visits his parents in Abingdon, Oxfordshire. His mother is shocked by his appearance. 'He looked as if he had been living on the streets for weeks. He had white, dry skin all over his forehead and in his eyebrows and on his eyelids. He was just so ill that he never went back.'

The transition is tough. The first thing he says when he enters their home is: 'I smell gas.' They have to turn off the supply, which means no central heating, and Jill has to cook on a portable electric hob in a lean-to alongside the kitchen that is partly open to the elements. The task they now have is to find him somewhere permanent to live, and an income to survive on.

In late 2004, with his parents' support, Mark applies for disability living allowance, to help with his extra day-to-day costs as a disabled person. His claim is rejected, and he lodges an appeal, prepared by his mother and Oxfordshire Welfare Rights. His consultant psychiatrist confirms in a letter that he is 'severely disabled with long standing personality difficulties' and concludes: 'I have no doubt that he is unable to provide for his own personal daily care without a considerable amount of direct help currently.'

Jill tells the tribunal Mark 'needs help in virtually all aspects of daily living' and 'is not a good judge of the level of support that he requires.' The appeal is successful, and the ruling eases his financial problems, paying for some of his extra costs, such as his frequent taxis. He has also been found eligible for incapacity benefit, thanks in part to the detailed information about his support needs provided by his mother. With eligibility established for both DLA and incapacity benefit, for the first time in his life, Mark has enough money to live on.

Jill hears of a scheme run by a local housing association that allows disabled people on benefits to buy a shared ownership house. Mark's parents and the housing association, Advance, both contribute capital, with the monthly mortgage to be paid from his income support payments.

In late 2005, after months of hard work, his parents find a small house in the village of Bampton. On moving day, in January, they arrive with Mark's belongings, but the moment he opens the door, he says: 'I can't stay here. There's this terrible smell.' They had asked the previous owners not to put any air fresheners in the house, but there they are in the electric sockets. They return to Abingdon with all his furniture.

His parents pay for the house to be cleaned, with the walls and ceilings washed twice without using chemicals. When they return to Bampton, Mark says it is no better, but his mother tells him: 'Mark, this is your home, you are going to stay here.' He decides the smell is less of a problem in the kitchen-dining-room, so that is where they put his bed. For the next seven years, the rest of the house is used for storage.

* * *

The first hint of the trouble ahead comes in October 2012, when Jill receives a letter warning that the government is reassessing disabled people on incapacity benefit for the new ESA and that this could lead to their benefits being cut, and, they warn, 'their home could be at risk'.

Jill writes to Mark, warning him that he could lose his home. 'To avoid this happening,' she writes, 'you need to tell them clearly and emphatically what your problems are and why you would not be able to work.' She passes on details of organisations that could support him, and says she would be happy to help 'if you would be willing to accept it'. She stresses that, if he is found fit for work, 'you can appeal against it'.

By the time the Gants receive the letter, Mark has already been sent – and has completed and returned – an ESA50 questionnaire. He is part of the huge group of claimants being reassessed through the work capability assessment process.

Mark has played down his impairments, but he has alerted DWP and Atos to some of the challenges he faces. He says he has 'multiple chemical allergies, migraines symptoms and nausea and depression' which 'affect where I go and also travel'. He describes his acute social anxieties as 'basically shyness and lack self-confidence at times'. Thanks to evidence from his GP about his panic attacks, Atos agrees to visit Mark in his own home.

On 2 February 2013, an Atos doctor visits Mark in Bampton. The ESA85 form* subsequently filled in by the doctor is completed

* The ESA85 form is a medical report form completed by an assessor following a face-to-face assessment.

in an untidy scrawl of capital letters that in places is impossible to read. There is little detail. In the summary, the doctor says Mark states that he has anxiety and depression and multiple chemical sensitivity but that the MCS is 'not causing functional problems'. He mentions Mark's past alcohol and cannabis misuse, that he has a 'normal typical day routine', and that his 'observed behaviour was unremarkable'. He concludes that Mark can be assessed next time at a medical assessment centre, rather than at home, because 'customer can use public transport'.

Mark appears to have told the doctor he is receiving no current treatment for his MCS, that his cannabis and alcohol problems are in the past ('teetotal for many years') and that he is receiving no anxiety medication. The doctor describes Mark as 'self-employed' and as living independently for six years. The report says he shops locally, sees a few friends, and 'does his own chores', but it does note that he receives DLA, before adding: 'No behavioural problems, no court cases; no other physical health problems.' On every activity, the doctor ticks the 'None of the above apply' box, including the sections on learning tasks, and the activity relating to planning, organisation, problem solving, prioritising or switching tasks. The 'coping with change' section is also ticked 'None of the above apply'. The doctor's conclusion is that work could be considered within three months because Mark has 'no significant functional problems'. The assessment appears to have taken just 20 minutes, with the report completed just 30 minutes later.

The doctor's conclusions are rubber-stamped by a DWP decision-maker, who decides Mark is fit for work. DWP later says this evaluation was made by a senior decision-maker with 'many years' experience.

There has been no attempt to secure the years of medical evidence that would have demonstrated Mark's impairments, and no attempt to contact any of the medical professionals who could have expanded on this evidence. There is no mention of the detailed account of his impairments Mark's mother wrote as part of his application for incapacity benefit in 2004. The decision-maker merely refers to 'anxiety and depression and allergy (multiple chemical sensitivity)'.

Although DWP later insists that the answers Mark provided in his ESA50 questionnaire did 'not suggest a significant level of functional impairment', it adds: 'Nevertheless DWP considers that the Healthcare Professional's report was not sufficiently detailed and the assessor did not take a thorough case history.'

A subsequent statement from Mark's GP, Dr Nicholas Ward, details some of the evidence that would have been available if requested. It includes Mark's time at the Churchill Clinic in 1995; his visits to a consultant psychiatrist in 1997; his daily suicidal thoughts in March 2003; his diagnosis of MCS in June 2004; descriptions of his addictive, obsessive behaviour, depression and anxiety, by a consultant psychiatrist in June 2004; a review by a consultant psychiatrist in January 2005 that suggested 'his rehabilitation would take years'; his description of 'low mood, social isolation' and 'an abnormal relationship with food' in May 2008; a consultation about his binge eating in April 2009; how his body mass index had continued to fall from 2010 to 2011; his request for a home assessment for DLA in September 2012 because he had panic attacks if he travelled to Oxford; and further discussions about his eating disorder in April 2013.

In April, Dr Ward writes a 'TO WHOM IT MAY CONCERN' letter – which Jill Gant will later describe as a 'definitive statement of Mark's health condition' – explaining that Mark is 'extremely unwell and absolutely unfit for any work whatsoever', mentioning his 'extremely low and very dangerous' body mass index of 14, and pleading: 'Mark is in no way fit to work and we are trying to arrange some emergency help for him. Please do not stop or reduce his benefits as this will have ongoing, significant impact on his mental health. He is simply not well enough to cope with this extra stress. His mental and medical condition is extremely serious.'

It is not clear what Mark does with this letter, but Dr Ward will say later that Mark told him that having his benefits removed had made him feel 'very, very unwell, that he felt very stressed' and 'didn't know how to cope with it'.

Despite efforts by the Bampton GP surgery to persuade Mark to attend a specialist eating disorder unit, he cancels the appointment.

His BMI at this stage is 14.1, which a clinical psychologist from the unit says is 'very low indeed for a male'. Mark speaks to Dr Ward on 3 May and says he has 'gained a few pounds and had been eating more protein and fish' but finds appointments 'extremely stressful' and says they would 'adversely affect his appetite and cause more weight loss'.

'I explained to him the extreme dangers of his weight loss and that there was serious risk of heart failure, renal failure, osteoporosis, sudden death etc,' Dr Ward wrote later. 'Mark said he understood these risks and accepted them.' Mark says that if anyone from the eating disorder unit or mental health services visits him at home, he will leave the area.

By now, the surgery is considering having Mark sectioned under the Mental Health Act, but Dr Ward decides that would probably cause him 'extreme distress' and the same outcome. On 6 May, Mark calls NHS 111, explains his weight loss and mentions that his GP says he needs mental health treatment. But he says he has made a mistake and hangs up.

Mark returns to the surgery on 24 May and his weight is recorded as 46.6 kg, but another GP says he needed to be weighed without his clothes on. He phones the surgery later to say he 'wished to be left alone as he was becoming increasingly stressed'. He returns to the surgery but will not enter the treatment room, saying he is 'extremely worried' about being institutionalised.

By 5 June, his weight has fallen to 43.2 kg (less than seven stone). Dr Ward wrote later: 'Mark telephoned me to indicate that he found it very stressful when he had been weighed that day ... He reiterated his belief that he could sort out the eating problem if he was left to his own devices.' He last speaks to Dr Ward on 11 July, when the GP again suggests he comes to the surgery to be properly weighed, and encourages him to increase his fluid intake during hot weather.

Although Mark will occasionally meet his sister Cathie for a cup of tea, or call for a chat, his contact with her has gradually reduced over the years, encouraged by the counsellor who advised him years earlier to develop independence from his family.

That changes in the spring of 2013. Mark suddenly begins to call Cathie. He claims he needs to see someone from Alcoholics Anonymous in Devon and needs a break because he is feeling 'rotten'. He makes repeated calls over the next two months. Some days he will phone between six and ten times, each time changing his mind or worrying that he has upset his sister.

Meanwhile, unknown to his family, he is losing more weight. Details gradually emerge about his financial problems. He is £500 in debt on his electricity bill. He agrees the family can pay this off. There is also a problem with his housing benefit, so the family contact Advance. Then he tells Cathie something else, that he has been seen by a doctor called 'Atos' but he has no idea why. 'I was very surprised as he never let anyone into his house,' says Cathie. 'I then realised he'd probably had his benefits cut off – possibly in April – and was in real trouble financially and just living off his DLA.'

An Advance housing officer, Jennifer Keeble, later tells Oxfordshire Coroner's office that Mark told her he was 'having trouble with the benefit people and he couldn't cope with the stress of dealing with it all, to the point that he would prefer to live on his DLA alone'. His housing benefit has been cut off, but Keeble manages to have it reinstated.

Mark tells Keeble he has had a visit from Atos and believes it is to do with his DLA. Keeble believes Mark has been placed in the ESA work-related activity group, and subsequently had his ESA removed because he failed to attend work-related sessions. She tells him he will need to complete a new ESA form. After answering just a few questions he says he can't cope and that DWP already has the information. Jill and Advance submit a new ESA application on Mark's behalf, with Advance hand-delivering it on 19 July to a member of jobcentre staff who knows Mark's case. The form is sent to one of DWP's regional benefit centres.

Jill waits to hear from DWP, but there is nothing. The department files the form and forgets about it. DWP tells the family later they should have submitted an ESA1 claim form, rather than an ESA50. By then it is too late.

Mark eventually agrees to accept £250 in cash in an envelope through Advance. They persuade him the money has come from his deceased grandparents. His family 'breathed a sigh of relief,' said Cathie. He now has money for food and as he is no longer phoning, they think he is OK. They have no idea about his drastic weight loss.

They later discover Mark had given most of the money to the vicar of Bampton, the Revd David Lloyd, to keep hold of. He had been worried about it coming from 'people who had died'. The vicar has known Mark since he moved to Bampton. Mark has occasionally asked him for a reference for voluntary jobs or to borrow 'a few pounds when he was in financial difficulties'. He always repays the money.

Revd Lloyd will later say he had seen Mark looking 'very gaunt in the face' and wearing several layers of clothing, despite the hot weather. 'It was obvious that he was painfully thin and unwell.' Mark assures the clergyman he has seen his GP. He will borrow a few pounds, pay some of it back and then borrow more. He eventually pays back the £50 he owes from the money his family has sent through Advance. Towards the end of July, he tells the vicar he is resolving his benefits problems.

On 26 July, Mark phones Revd Lloyd for the last time. He is in Bampton market square and isn't feeling well. He asks if he can drive him home. 'I took the car around and gave him a lift home,' the vicar would write later. 'He was still swathed in layers of clothes on a very hot day, but seemed quite lucid and got in and out of the car without help. He didn't want me to come into the house or take any further action.'

Meanwhile, Jill is understandably distracted. Her husband, Mark's step-father, is seriously ill. He dies on 2 August. Cathie soon begins to worry that she has not heard from her brother and debates whether to text Mark to let him know John has died. She decides it would upset him too much. John's funeral takes place on 7 August. Cathie talks to relatives about what to do, and decides to write Mark a text, but doesn't send it.

It is Cathie who is told about her brother's death on 9 August. She is told he has probably been dead for a while. Jill returns home on

10 August. Cathie visits her mother in Abingdon later that day to tell her that Mark has died.

* * *

The inquest takes place on 25 February 2014. A pathologist says Mark's body mass index was just 11.3. A body mass index of about 12 to 13 is 'generally considered potentially fatal'. It was 19.4 in 2009, 17.5 in 2011, and fell to 13.4 in May 2013. A BMI of 18.5 to 24.9 is considered healthy. The pathologist concludes that Mark probably died from a heart attack caused by his weight loss.

Both Jill and Cathie advocate for Mark in the inquest, attempting – without success – to show the coroner how crucial the loss of his benefits was in triggering the issues that caused his death.

Cathie manages to secure the crucial fact from Dr Ward that neither Atos nor DWP had asked him for information. The GP tells the inquest he believes 'something pushed him or affected him' in the months before he died and 'the only thing I can put my finger on was the pressure that he felt he was under when his benefits were removed'.

'And he certainly couldn't cope with that added pressure mentally,' the GP says, 'and I think it's a shame that he was put under that pressure, because he was too vulnerable to cope with it.'

Jill calmly tells the coroner she is convinced that the 'precipitating cause' of Mark's death was the loss of his benefits and 'the extreme stress' caused by the subsequent lack of money, which intensified his eating problems.

Cathie's written statement has also been clear: 'My judgement is that an already mentally ill and struggling man was tipped over the edge into further phobic/OCD behaviour which included food,' she writes. 'It's hard to say whether having no money caused him not to be able to eat properly for months or it made him so distressed that he couldn't get help when he needed it. Probably a toxic mix of the two – he wasn't well but he died prematurely and he would probably be alive today if they had not taken away his benefits in April.'

But the coroner ignores the evidence of Dr Ward, Cathie Wood, and Jill Gant, and suggests the money Mark's family sent him meant he had the resources to buy food if he wanted to. He says he cannot conclude that 'the loss of the benefits directly led to Mark starving to death'. Instead, he says he died through 'a natural cause and possibly a cardiac arrhythmia' to which his eating disorder and food phobia probably contributed.

When Jill asks if he will refer to a possible contribution of the removal of benefits, he tells her he is not 'in a position to say that' although he accepts Dr Ward's evidence 'about something pushing Mark over the edge'.

Both Jill and Cathie are outraged at the circumstances of Mark's death and frustrated with the coroner's failure to reference benefits in his verdict. Cathie speaks to the media after the inquest and says her brother was a 'sweet and gentle' person who 'didn't deserve to die'. She tells the *Oxford Mail*: 'Atos are completely to blame. If they had not evaluated him as normal he would have carried on in his own way and would not have died last summer.'[1]

She tells *The Guardian*:[2] 'I would like Iain Duncan Smith to stop talking about this as a moral crusade, and admit that this whole process of reassessing people for their benefits is a cost-cutting measure … This is not just someone being inconvenienced – this is a death.'

Cathie also talks to the *Mirror*.[3] 'When the police found him, there was very little food in the house, just half a banana and a tin of tuna,' she says. 'Anyone who knew Mark's complex problems would see he couldn't work … I'd like David Cameron and his government to be aware of the personal cost of their policies and how they are affecting real people and causing real heartache.'

DWP responds in typical fashion, with a spokesperson offering the following – deeply misleading – statement: 'A decision on whether someone is well enough to work is taken following a thorough assessment and after consideration of all the supporting medical evidence from the claimant's GP or medical specialist.'

The following month, DWP admits Mark should not have been found fit for work. The decision comes in the week that Atos announces it is pulling out early from its five-year contract to deliver the WCA.

On 27 November, Cathie joins Gill Thompson at a public meeting organised by Oxfordshire Green Party in David Cameron's Witney constituency. It is titled: 'Austerity Kills on David Cameron's Doorstep: Why Did Mark Wood and David Clapson Starve to Death?' Cathie tells the meeting her brother's death was a direct result of being declared fit for work, and that he and others have been 'sacrificed to benefit cuts'.

Jill writes to her MP, Nicola Blackwood. Looking back, she praises Blackwood for being 'absolutely punctilious in making sure that my questions were answered' and ensuring she secured a meeting with the minister for disabled people, Mark Harper. Jill tells Harper it is 'totally and utterly unjust' that the assessment process does not ensure there is a medical report from the healthcare professionals that know the claimant.

She experiences Harper's attitude as 'cold'. 'He didn't seem to listen to or engage with the story or the basis of the justice of the case, and didn't seem moved by it at all,' she tells me. Once again, the need to ensure further medical evidence in cases like Mark's is dismissed. When she finds out later that a coroner made a similar demand in early 2010, following the death of Stephen Carré, she is 'horrified and angry'.

Years later, she tells me a change of policy to ensure this kind of further medical evidence is provided with each claim would give her some 'closure'. 'Nothing would make Mark's death OK, but something good would have come out of it so that other people wouldn't suffer the same appalling inequity,' she says.

* * *

On 14 October 2015, Jill gives evidence in London to the UN committee on the rights of persons with disabilities, as part of its investigation into DWP's breaches of the UN disability convention.

Jill and Cathie are determined that Mark is not just remembered for the way he died. Jill arranges an exhibition of his watercolours, cartoons, short stories, photography, and poetry at Oxford Town Hall. The theme is Mark's love of the environment. In a pamphlet, Jill describes her son's 'rich visual, musical and verbal imagination', and how he was 'determined to express his talent in the pursuit of his passion to save the world'.

His writing and cartoons are quirky, imaginative, and amusing, with many featuring a talking cat called Leonard. The theme is always saving the planet from ecological disaster. He was, says his mother, 'a very creative person who was passionate about nature and highly sensitive to the damage that was being done to wildlife and our planetary home'.

Jill blames Mark's death on an attitude that 'people on benefit are scroungers and that we really can't support too many of them'. The government's language, she says, conveys a hostility to claimants. 'It's a kind of resentment,' she says. 'I can't understand it myself, I can't understand why there's such hostility to dependent people.'

14

The Death of David Barr

August 2013. David's dad, a bus driver, also called David, has driven his son back to his flat in Glenrothes. His parents are divorced, his dad living in nearby Leven, and his mum also in Glenrothes, a post-1945 new town about 30 miles north of Edinburgh across the Firth of Forth.

His dad knows there are letters and papers scattered across the floor of his son's flat, so he has brought folders with him to organise and keep them safe. He has brought his son a bacon roll and a newspaper and made him a cup of tea. While he is sorting out the papers and chatting away, he sees his son's hands are shaking.

'Dad, can I talk to you?' he says.

'Look, you'll get better, it will be OK. I'll take you down your mum's and you'll get some tea,' his dad replies, and gives him a tenner. He would normally give him more, but it's all he has. David notices his son has written a poem on the wall of the living room:

Lovely lady of the moon
Bring me money sometime soon
Do not harm any on its way
Give me money because I cannot stay
Of fair amount will be good
Thank you
lady of the moon

28 years and fifty days
David William Barr

His age – 28 years and 50 days – shows he had written it earlier that day, 23 August. His dad asks him why he has written it on the wall.

'I liked it, dad,' he says.

When his dad has finished clearing up, David tells him: 'Aye, dad, you've done a good job.'

They drive to his mum's house and arrive at about 5.30pm. As his dad gets back in his car, David says: 'I'll see you when I see you, dad.'

'He knew I hated that expression, because it means nothing,' says David snr. 'And that was the last time I saw him.'

* * *

David's mum, Maureen, remembers her son always wanting to be up and about. 'He had a couple of friends, and once they got together they were away,' she told me. 'We lived in Leven at the time, so we were near the beach. He liked being down the beach and other places.'

David travelled a lot growing up. His dad, originally from Belfast, joined a Scottish army regiment at 15, and met Maureen in Scotland. He was posted to Cyprus, Germany, and Oman, and his son often joined him there during the holidays. 'Every time he came to Germany, we always bought him a bike,' says his dad. 'And me and him, we would go off some place. He was a tough wee bugger. He had some determination. If he put his mind to something, it was done.'

Back in Scotland, he loved football and used to cycle for miles in the countryside. His parents split up when he was about ten, and he shuttled between their homes, often staying with his mum during the week and his dad at weekends, but sometimes visiting his dad off the school bus before heading to his mum's.

He was 16 when he left school, and for the next ten years or so found work around Fife, as a casual labourer, picking fruit and vegetables, working on construction jobs. He was a hard worker. His dad eventually found him a job cleaning buses, and for a time it went well, and he had steady money. But he gave up his flat to move in with his girlfriend, and when they broke up weeks later, he was left shuttling between his parents' houses or sleeping on friends' floors.

The bus job with Stagecoach was 4pm until 2am and he began to miss days, and sometimes left work before his shift finished. Eventually, in 2011, he quit after being disciplined for missing a day's work. Within a few hours, he asked for the job back, but they wouldn't take him.

He had been living in a series of 'scatter flats', temporary accommodation for those on the waiting-list for a permanent council home. His last flat, in Craigellachie Court, is in a quiet cul-de-sac intended for older and disabled people. The walls are stained brown with nicotine, and his dad helps him redecorate, and weeds the back garden. His dad asks the council for furniture, a fridge and cooker, because every time David moves home – as he has done repeatedly – he loses everything, apart from whatever he can carry in a small backpack.

His deteriorating mental health leads to several run-ins with the law, including a minor assault, and a fine for setting light to a wheelie-bin after a feud with a neighbour. There is another fine after he lights a small fire in the back garden of his flat in Leven, and then falls asleep inside as the embers set light to his shed. When the police arrive, they find him still asleep. He explains he had drunk a bottle of wine and taken a sleeping tablet and curled up on the couch to sleep.

For a short period from July 2011, David has been able to claim employment and support allowance (ESA) after losing his job, but that stops in October 2011 after he fails to return forms he had been sent. For the next couple of years, he has to rely on jobseeker's allowance. His debts grow. His parents help him out with cash, but neither of them know of his financial problems.

In July 2012, he self-harms, and tells his psychiatrist about this incident and a suicide attempt a couple of weeks earlier. He tries again to claim ESA in 2012, but his claim is rejected because he fails to attend a face-to-face assessment. He applies a third time in 2013, and this time he fails to return the ESA50 questionnaire. Because of his mental health history, the claim is kept open, and Atos tells him to attend a face-to-face assessment in nearby Kirkcaldy on 22 May.

His mother travels with him on the train, but he attends the assessment alone. His dad had bought him some new trainers, and his clothes are clean. The assessor, a physiotherapist, describes him as 'well kempt' and 'neatly dressed' and says he 'did not appear to be trembling'. In his report, he notes that David last attempted suicide just six weeks earlier, has occasional thoughts of harming himself, has previously tried to take his own life, and 'is anxious all the time'.

There is further evidence of his mental distress. 'Always sleeps poorly due to thinking about things. He washes his hands all the time. He gets paranoid that people are watching him and people are listening to him.' He notes that David is waiting to be transferred to a new psychiatric team after moving home in January. Before that, he was being seen by both a psychiatric nurse and a psychiatrist.

The assessor also notes those things David says he can do, such as dressing, making meals, shopping, and that he will go for walks with a friend in the country, visit the library, read books, watch TV, and listen to music. The assessor then adds: 'A last minute change in his GP appointment could spark a panic attack, he is not sure.' The assessor describes David's mood in the assessment as 'irritable and impatient, but I mostly found him disinterested', adding: 'Overall his mental state exam was largely unremarkable.'

In the 'personalised summary statement' – despite David insisting on standing against the wall during the assessment – the assessor states: 'I found his condition history inconsistent and his medication dosage inconsistent. His typical day and mental state exam overall do not support significant restrictions.'

He concludes: 'The evidence, including the condition history and mental state examination, does not suggest that the client's Mental Health Problem would mean there would be a substantial risk to the mental or physical health of any person if they were found capable of work or work related activity.' The assessment lasts just 35 minutes, and the assessor takes just another 18 minutes to write his report.

DWP twice attempts to speak to David. On both occasions – 11 and 12 June – they call his mum's house, but do not manage to speak to him. They make no attempt to follow up with a letter, and do not ask him to call them back.

A week later, on 19 June, David is told the result of his assessment by letter. Despite the errors, inconsistencies and alarming gaps in the assessment report, the DWP decision-maker repeatedly states that she has 'weighed the evidence and the [physiotherapist's] evidence carries more weight'. She says there is 'no evidence of substantial risk' and no evidence that David is 'unable to cope with day to day living'. The report, she concludes, is 'appropriate', 'complete', and 'comprehensive'. David would have needed 15 points to be found eligible for ESA. He is awarded six. He is told he is fit for work.

On 28 June, David fills in a form and attaches a letter appealing the decision. He tells DWP: *'I am writing to let you know that I disagree with your decision that I am fit for work! I have Serious mental health problems that prevent me from doing everyday tasks which means I cannot at this moment in time be able to work. I did try and explain this to the medical examiner at the time.'*

On 8 July, David is interviewed by police on the Forth Road Bridge, after he is found 'drunk and incapable' and 'unsteady on his feet', looking over the railings into the water below. He tells them he is walking to Edinburgh, about eight miles away. The officers conclude he is not considering taking his own life, and they take no further action.

On 17 July, someone from DWP calls David's mother's home, but leaves no message. There is no further attempt to contact David. The DWP civil servant who decides his appeal concludes that the Atos assessor's evidence is more believable than David's, repeatedly writing: 'I have weighed the evidence and the [physiotherapist's] evidence carries more weight.'

She writes: 'While Mr Barr reports occasional thoughts of self harm he has not been seen by a Community Psychiatric Nurse since moving in January 2013.' This information is wrong: the assessment report makes it clear he saw his CPN in April 2013. The civil servant ignores David's disclosure of a recent suicide attempt, just six weeks before he was assessed. The assessment report, the DWP civil servant concludes, was 'appropriate', 'complete', and 'comprehensive'.

On 25 July, David receives a letter telling him he will need to pay more than £90 a month in council tax for the next few months. The next day, he receives the papers he needs to take his case to tribunal. On 19 August, he receives a bank statement that says he has just 36p in his account.

'I noticed the last six months he was going downhill,' David Barr snr says in 2022 when I visit him at his home in Leven. We had spoken several times on the phone in the previous six years, but this is the first time we have met. The grief appears just as raw, but as on previous occasions when we'd spoken, he seems grateful for the chance to talk about his much-loved son.

In the spring and summer of 2013, David jnr has been drinking too much, in combination with his medication: sleeping pills, anti-depressants, anti-psychotics. He has been seen in a bar in Glenrothes with his head on the bar. His dad picks him up, takes him home, puts him to bed.

He has been moved to a health centre on the other side of town after staff at the surgery lose patience with him missing early appointments he sleeps through because of medication side-effects. The transfer means he drifts away from the regular support he needs, although he is still seeing his community psychiatric nurse.

His dad tries to keep an eye on him through friends in Glenrothes. When David snr goes on holiday, he gives money to the barman at the Station Hotel and asks him to give it to his son £30 at a time.

On 14 August, England are playing Scotland in a friendly at Wembley and the two of them are watching the match in a bar. David notices his son's eyes rolling in his head. He insists he is OK. He's only had a couple of drinks. Later that evening, his son walks past a bus driver without showing his pass. His dad apologises and takes him home in a taxi. 'I couldn't even trust him to get on the bus,' he said later. The driver reports the incident to the police liaison officer at the bus company, Stagecoach, and the police contact David snr. David tells his dad he shouldn't have spoken to the police. 'The police are after me,' he says, 'they're always watching me.'

'He always thought somebody was following him,' David snr told me. 'It was getting worse and worse and worse. Some days he looked fine, but he would also hallucinate and tell me he was being chased.'

David loves jazz and poetry, and visiting the Edinburgh Festival fringe and watching acts on the street, even if he can't afford to attend many shows, and he often takes the bus from Glenrothes, across the Forth Road Bridge and into the city. Earlier in the week, David had told his dad: 'I won't be here much longer.' His dad replied: 'Don't talk like that, you'll be alright. Don't do anything silly. Promise you won't do anything silly.' His son didn't answer.

His mum remembers him sitting at the computer for hours, listening to David Icke's conspiracy theories. Her husband, David's step-dad, would hide the computer. 'I tried to get him to talk about it, but he wouldn't,' says Maureen. 'It was as though he knew it was wrong.' It was around this time his mental health began to deteriorate, she says.

Eventually, a psychiatrist and a psychiatric nurse attempt to persuade Maureen, a nurse herself, to allow her son to be taken into hospital. 'I didn't think David was as ill as they thought he was,' Maureen told me. She asked her son, and he said no.

She now regrets not pushing for him to be admitted. She remembers how lonely her son was. 'He was staying here a lot of the time. We had got him a house not far from here, but he didn't really want to stay there. Thinking back now, it breaks my heart. He would always take the dog with him to keep him company. He was a lovely boy. I wish I had kept him here because he just hated being on his own.'

David did not enjoy having his picture taken but one photograph sits on the mantelpieces of both his mum's and his dad's homes. It was taken by his dad at a family barbecue. His son is frowning, anxious, his hair covered by a dark blue beanie.

On 23 August, Maureen cooks a meal. David eats something but doesn't want to sit down. He tells her he is going to Edinburgh. 'I said to remember to be back before the last bus.' She gives him £10 for the fare. David says goodbye and leaves. But he returns and asks for a painkiller. He says he doesn't feel well. She suggests he stays home, but he insists he wants to go to Edinburgh. He leaves at about 6pm for the five-minute walk to the bus station.

He catches a bus to the Ferrytoll park and ride, about a mile from the Forth Road Bridge. The 20-mile journey, along the tree-lined A92 dual carriageway, is bleak and beautiful. As the bus approaches Ferrytoll, the majestic Forth Road Bridge looms in the distance.

David's body is pulled into an RNLI lifeboat at about 8.15pm. He is still conscious and breathing and tells them his name, although they mishear it as Dave Marr. Before they arrive at the South Queensferry pier, he goes into cardiac arrest. Paramedics administer CPR as the ambulance speeds to Edinburgh Royal Infirmary with a police escort. David is pronounced dead on arrival at the hospital.

* * *

David's dad reads the report of the Atos assessor and is determined to seek justice. He contacts the *Daily Record*. He tells reporter Craig McDonald his ex-wife has been left 'completely broken', and is now in hospital, having barely eaten since he died.

David tells the *Record*: 'They said David was fit for work but, in fact, he was fit for hospital. I'm in no doubt this matter was the final straw. I would say they are 90 per cent to blame for him taking his life. I just hope something can be done so no-one else has to go through this.'

DWP delivers another cold, unrepentant statement, telling the *Record*: 'Through a series of independent reviews and by working with medical experts and charities, we have considerably improved the work capability assessment process since 2010.'

Just a month or so later, DWP reverses its decision and admits David should have been eligible for ESA, although it still insists he should have been placed in the work-related activity group. The department eventually pays his family the nearly £3,000 extra he should have been receiving between October 2011 and 23 August 2013, the day he died.

David complains to DWP. About a year after David's death, two senior DWP officials visit his house to 'explain' what happened.

Maureen is there, and her sister and brother-in-law. The DWP officials are there for 90 minutes. David asks them: 'If it had been your son, would you have acted in the same way?'

He tells me later: 'They couldn't answer. They thought they had all the answers, but I said, "Don't preach to me about your system when you know it's wrong." I gave it to them with both barrels and they walked out of there with their tails between their legs, but it didn't bring my son back.'

He pushes the procurator fiscal – the Scottish equivalent of a coroner – to carry out a full investigation, known as a fatal accident inquiry. David argues that DWP's actions caused his son to take his own life. In July 2014, DWP passes its own internal review into David's death to the procurator fiscal.

On 11 December 2014, the procurator fiscal depute writes to David, although he does not receive the letter until 6 February 2015. She appears to have taken everything DWP has told her at face value. She says: 'The WCA remains the subject of continuous review and refinement by a number of different independent routes and it appears therefore that a Fatal Accident Inquiry would not assist in monitoring and reviewing this process which is already underway.'

She adds: 'This case has also been considered by our National [Scottish Fatalities Investigation Unit] and they conclude that it would be difficult in terms of the legal test, on the balance of probabilities, to make the necessary link between the decision of the DWP and David's decision to take his life.'

He objects, but a Scottish government lawyer rejects his appeal. There will be no fatal accident inquiry.

David also supports an attempt by Black Triangle to persuade Scottish police to investigate Iain Duncan Smith and Chris Grayling. Black Triangle's co-founder, John McArdle, submits a dossier of evidence, including reports on the death of David Barr.

McArdle believes the two politicians are guilty of the Scottish criminal offence of wilful neglect of duty by a public official, because they failed to improve the work capability assessment process in 2010 after being warned by Tom Osborne – following the death of Stephen Carré – that its flaws risked causing future deaths. The attempt fails, with Scottish criminal agencies deciding in late 2016 to take no further action.[1]

When I first speak to David in 2016, he insists the 'fit for work' finding was 'definitely' the trigger for his son's suicide. 'It was all in the brown envelopes, the paperwork,' he says. 'Every time I've seen Iain Duncan Smith on the TV I've had to walk out or turn it off,' he says. 'I hate the man with a vengeance. If he ever came up here to Fife or Edinburgh, you'd better keep him away from me. I'd spit at him, or worse, I'd throw an egg at him. He knows what's going on and he does nothing about it. I want those two, Chris Grayling and Iain Duncan Smith, to be accountable for what they've done.'

I tell him about the Stephen Carré prevention of future deaths report, and its call for action on further medical evidence, three years before David died. He is shocked. 'It's gone on and they've done nothing about it. The ministers in charge of everything should have sorted something out, stopped it, changed it, redirected it.' He compares the WCA to a dangerously faulty vehicle. 'If we had a defective bus, you wouldn't let it go in the road,' he says, 'you'd be up for manslaughter. These people should be taken to court.'

15
The Death of Ms DE

As evidence slowly emerges of the damage being caused by the work capability assessment, I catch Peter Lilley after a fringe event at the Conservative conference in Manchester in October 2013. He tells me he has 'no objection in principle' to the WCA, and does not believe it is significantly different from his own all work test. 'If they have improved it, so much the better,' he says. 'Generally, they built on what I did rather than scrapped it. Generally, I take it as a degree of endorsement.'

He denies that parts of the insurance industry have spent two decades lobbying the government to tighten eligibility. 'I don't think we envisaged this being a sort of signal that everybody should get private insurance. I don't remember thinking about that,' he says. 'It shouldn't be a signal.'

I ask if he remembers bringing in John LoCascio to advise the government on the assessment process. 'When I was secretary of state?' he asks. 'Maybe, I'm not denying it, but I certainly don't remember. If you tell me it happened, it happened, but I have absolutely no recollection. If there had been a rumpus about it at the time I would have thought I would remember.'

Maybe he had forgotten the coverage in *Private Eye* in 1995, the paper written by LoCascio and Aylward in August 1995, and the briefing he was given by DSS civil servants in March 1996 telling him how to respond if asked about LoCascio's appointment.

When we exchange emails in early 2023 he says again that he has 'no recollection of employing Unum or John LoCascio, though maybe we did'.

* * *

11 October 2013. DPAC co-founders Debbie Jolly and Linda Burnip, with legal support from solicitor Louise Whitfield, meet Jorge Araya, secretary to the UN committee on the rights of persons with disabilities. They persuade him to investigate allegations of 'systematic and grave' violations of disabled people's human rights, focusing on policies introduced by DWP ministers. The UK becomes the first country to face such a high-level inquiry.

But Labour is not listening. The following day, Rachel Reeves, Labour's new shadow work and pensions secretary, vows her party will be tougher on welfare than the coalition.[1] 'Nobody should be under any illusions that they are going to be able to live a life on benefits under a Labour government,' says Reeves.

Four months after the death of David Clapson, employment minister Esther McVey issues a press release.[2] She wants to end the 'something for nothing' culture. She brags about new figures which show jobseeker's allowance claimants have had their payments suspended 580,000 times in the nine months since 'tougher rules' were introduced in October 2012.

'People who are in a job know that if they don't play by the rules or fail to turn up in the morning, there might be consequences, so it's only right that people on benefits should have similar responsibilities,' says McVey.

The following month, Dr Paul Litchfield, chief medical officer for BT Group, publishes the fourth independent review of the WCA.[3] He says only 34 of the 49 recommendations made by Professor Harrington over his three reviews have been implemented in full. But there is no mention of the secret reviews that – it will later emerge – are carried out by DWP civil servants when a claimant's death has been linked to DWP. And there is no mention of the Stephen Carré prevention of future deaths report. The words 'death' and 'suicide' do not appear in Litchfield's report.

* * *

Today, more than twelve years after she died on 31 December 2011, the identity of Ms DE remains unknown.

She was in her early 50s. She had worked in several jobs, including in the financial sector, and had 'a very difficult time' between 2006 and 2010, largely due to stress in her NHS clerical job, which eventually she quit. She was out of work for the last 21 months of her life. She was divorced, with one teenage son who lived with her ex-husband but saw his mum often. She had been in a new relationship for several years and was planning to marry her fiancé in mid-2012. She owned her own home, which had been re-mortgaged, and had been diagnosed with depression and anxiety. She had been prescribed an anti-depressant and lithium, which, a report would say later, indicated that her doctors found her condition 'difficult to treat'. She also had physical health problems and had been signed off work for her depression. She had several friends she saw regularly, some of them through a local church. She also did some volunteer work with teenagers.

Her first contact with a psychiatrist was in 1985, and in 1992 she became an outpatient of Dr A, a consultant psychiatrist. She first claimed incapacity benefit in 2007 and had three periods claiming the benefit that totalled nearly three years.

In July 2011 she was caught up in the three-year programme to reassess incapacity benefit claimants for the new employment and support allowance (ESA), just a few months after Chris Grayling launched the 'migration' process against the advice of Professor Malcolm Harrington. She had been receiving incapacity benefit (IB) for more than a year, but Dr A would say later she 'had been doing well' and was hoping to return to work.

She would later tell a welfare rights adviser she had never received the ESA50 questionnaire, which would have enabled her to describe the impact of her health conditions on her ability to work. Atos would later insist it sent her the questionnaire on 4 August and attempts to contact her by phone had failed.

Atos decided that, based on her original IB claim, there was little evidence to suggest she would qualify for ESA, so decided not to seek further medical evidence from her GP or Dr A. It went ahead with a face-to-face assessment on 26 October, carried out by 'an experienced doctor'. It lasted an hour. The only information the doctor had in advance about Ms DE was one word: 'depression'. There was no questionnaire. There were no medical reports from her GP or Dr A. She was awarded zero points.

In DWP's subsequent report, based on the assessment, a decision-maker stated that Ms DE was able to shower most days, 'manages to do her housework and does it in stages and usually completes it if getting visitors' and could 'manage stairs by holding on to the rails'. Once a week, she drove 'to the local shop, church, bible study group and drives to her voluntary work'.

The DWP decision-maker decided Ms DE was fit for work. She would have to claim jobseeker's allowance, and her income would fall by £26.75 a week to £67.50. On 9 December, DWP made two unsuccessful attempts to phone her, but left no messages. DWP sent her two letters, notifying her of the decision and telling her that her ESA would stop on 12 January. She was told she had received zero points in all 17 'functional areas' of the assessment.

She called her psychiatrist and GP. She was 'very distressed'. Dr A put her in touch with a welfare rights officer based at his hospital. The adviser told her she believed the decision would be overturned when DWP received letters from her psychiatrist and GP.

When she heard how sharply her benefits would be reduced, Ms DE became 'very upset'. 'She had been crying and saying that she didn't know how she was going to manage,' said the adviser later. 'She was extremely worried about how she would pay her mortgage.'

On the appeal form, Ms DE told DWP: 'I have both physical and mental health problems which impact greatly on each other. I feel the medical just focussed on my physical health though. I have found going from being an independent working woman to being on benefits extremely hard and has made my depression worse. My heart problems are still being investigated ... My health problems affect all activities of daily living.'

In a letter to support her appeal, Dr A said Ms DE was, at present, 'totally incapable of work'. Dr A spoke to her again four days later, and saw her on 22 December. She spoke to Dr A's registrar on 29 December. She denied any thoughts of suicide. Two days later, on

New Year's Eve, Ms DE was found dead at her house, 13 days before her ESA was due to be stopped.

Three months later, the associate medical director of the NHS board responsible for Ms DE wrote to the Mental Welfare Commission for Scotland. He said it should examine the case, because his colleagues felt changes in the benefits system were 'having a major adverse effect on their patients' and it might be helpful to 'look more closely into the circumstances to see whether any lessons could be learned'. The commission had heard similar concerns from 'service users, carers and professionals across Scotland'. It launched an inquiry.

Dr A tells the commission that both he and Ms DE's GP felt they should have been contacted by DWP. He is 'unaware of any other possible precipitants [apart from the WCA process] which could have contributed to her decision to take her own life'.

The GP had written a letter strongly in support of her appeal, stating that the assessment had 'dented her confidence and caused a worsening of depressive symptoms … and as such at present she is certainly unfit for work'. He, too, can think of no reason for her to take her own life, other than the reassessment. Subsequent reviews find no fault with the healthcare provided to Ms DE.

A friend describes how she met Ms DE while running parenting courses for a charity. Ms DE became a volunteer and started attending the same church as her friend, who says Ms DE became 'very worried' about how she would cope financially after being found fit for work.

A DWP civil servant tells the commission he has not identified 'any deficiencies in the DWP processes in this case', or in the Atos report, although he has identified some 'missed opportunities'. He has recommended DWP's guidance on vulnerable claimants should be 're-publicised' among staff, although Ms DE herself had not been regarded as vulnerable.

The Atos doctor who assessed Ms DE provides the 'personalised summary statement' she completed: 'She has depression, she regularly gets reviewed by psychiatry. She was started on mood stabilisers last year … She was timid at interview but otherwise her mental state appeared normal and despite her regular review by psychiatrist there is no evidence that she has a significant disability of mental health function.'

The commission is 'surprised' by this paragraph, as Ms DE 'had been seen by a consultant psychiatrist over the course of a 20 year period, was being frequently reviewed and was prescribed significant medication'. The doctor does not deny Ms DE had a mental health condition, just that there was no 'functional' impact. Mansel Aylward, John LoCascio, and their biopsychosocial model disciples would have approved. Atos and the DWP insist they made no errors.

As part of its inquiry, the commission surveys Scottish psychiatrists. Of the 56 who reply and have patients who have undergone a WCA, three-quarters say they have not been asked for their opinion by either Atos or DWP, while 96 per cent (all but two) say their patients were left 'distressed' by the process.

Two-fifths of those surveyed have at least one patient who has self-harmed following a WCA – partly because of the assessment process or the outcome – and seven of them (13 per cent) say at least one patient has attempted to take their own life, partly again because of the assessment. Two of the 56 say a patient has succeeded in taking their own life. One patient with a psychotic illness has 'incorporated the assessment process into his system of delusions, leading him to believe that he was being followed by the DWP'. More than a third say at least one of their patients has been admitted to hospital because of the WCA.

The commission's report concludes: 'We think that medical reports should be routinely obtained for individuals with a mental illness, learning disability or related condition entering the assessment process.'[4] It also says a DWP decision-maker should consider 'at least two distinct sources of information'. It calls for a review of how the WCA assesses people with mental distress.

DWP officials visit the commission and say they are keen to work with them on improvements to the WCA. But after they return to London, something changes. When the department releases its official response, it is complacent, claimant-blaming, defensive, and evasive, despite promising minor improvements and to trial limited changes. It says it remains 'committed to keeping [our] processes for collecting further evidence under constant review'. As for claimants with mental distress, like Ms DE, it believes that 'overall the WCA works as intended'.

Commenting on DWP's response, the commission says: 'We will continue to argue that the mental health information available in Ms DE's case was insufficient for such an important decision.'

If there had been a suicide linked to the provision of mental health services, the government would have expected a lengthy and probing review. The NHS is expected to have a duty of candour when a patient dies. But when a death is linked to DWP, the department takes every possible step to hide, confuse, obscure, and mislead.

16

DWP, Peer Reviews, and Weaponising Time

Throughout 2012, 2013, and 2014, local newspapers – and occasionally nationals – had been reporting on inquests and accounts from families of how their relatives had died after being wrongly found fit for work. But it isn't until the summer of 2014 that I begin to ask myself what the government knows about these deaths, what records it keeps, and how it responds to such tragedies.

I ask DWP through a freedom of information request what records it keeps 'of deaths that have been found to be connected to, or linked to, or partially caused by, the withdrawal or non-payment of disability benefits … from the person who has died' and 'how these deaths are collected, and how many such deaths there have been for each of the years 2004–2013'.

DWP replies on 22 September: 'The specific information requested is not held by the Department.' DWP is denying that it keeps any such records. This, it will soon emerge, is untrue.

Days later, when I question the minister for disabled people, Mark Harper, at the Conservative Party conference, he says he does not 'accept the premise' that DWP should collect and analyse reports that suggest a disabled person's death could have been linked to the non-payment or withdrawal of benefits. But this is contradicted the following week by a coalition colleague, the Liberal Democrat pensions minister Steve Webb, who tells me at his own party conference that 'when cases come up, clearly when the department becomes aware of cases through the media, they do get looked at.'[1]

Following this admission, DWP's press office finally confesses that the department does investigate some benefit-related deaths, saying: 'Where it is appropriate, we undertake reviews into individual cases but we do not accept the argument of those who seek to politicise people's deaths by linking them inaccurately to welfare policy.' (Neither I nor any other journalist had picked up on the references in the Ms DE report to a so-called 'peer review' process.)

I submit a fresh freedom of information request, which produces an admission that DWP has in fact carried out '60 peer reviews following the death of a customer' since February 2012 (it later amends this to 49 deaths and another eleven serious incidents). But DWP refuses to release any details about these reviews, claiming section 123 of the Social Security Administration Act (SSAA) 1992 makes it an offence for a DWP employee to disclose any information relating to a particular person without lawful authority (ie, the permission of the work and pensions secretary).

Information continues to trickle out. In February 2015, DWP admits that 40 of the 49 peer reviews were carried out following a suicide or apparent suicide. My news agency, Disability News Service (DNS), begins a lengthy battle with DWP to secure information from these peer reviews. The stumbling block is section 123, even though the information could be released if Iain Duncan Smith gave permission. Instead, he and subsequent work and pensions secretaries do everything they can to prevent any details of the fatal consequences of their policies being made public.

I ask DWP to reconsider its decision, suggesting it redacts any identifying information. DWP says this would still engage section 123. I lodge a complaint with the Information Commissioner's Office.

In October 2014, I learn from a researcher that the company set to take over the WCA contract from Atos has a 'chilling' record of incompetence, discrimination, and alleged fraud in the US.[2]

DWP's preferred bidder is US outsourcing giant Maximus. The previous year, US government auditors had found that all but $2 million of $41.4 million claimed by the state of Wisconsin – on advice from Maximus – had been 'improperly claimed' under Medicaid, the US healthcare insurance programme for those on low incomes. Maximus was reportedly paid a fee based on how much additional revenue the state collected. Concerns about its activities in the US date back more than 20 years. Maximus insists it has successfully run Welfare to Work and other programmes in more than 40 US states and around the world, including running more than 100 employment centres in the UK – where it is a Work Programme provider – and in Australia and Canada.

In November, Paul Litchfield publishes the fifth and final independent review of the work capability assessment.[3] He makes 28 recommendations but concludes that the WCA needs 'a period of stability', because although it is 'by no means perfect … there is no better replacement that can be pulled off the shelf'.

Rather than calling for significant reform, following so many deaths, he calls on the government to investigate 'as a matter of urgency' why there has been a substantial increase in the proportion of claimants placed in the ESA support group, for those who do not need to carry out any work-related activity. He suggests this might be due to increased use of ESA regulation 35.

Regulation 35 – seen as a safety net by many campaigners – states that a claimant should be placed in the ESA support group, rather than the work-related activity group (WRAG), if placing them in the WRAG would pose 'a substantial risk' to their 'mental or physical health'. DWP, and DSS before it, had tried repeatedly to remove this safety net, but these attempts had been defeated by the courts and its own advisory committee.

By now, disabled activists, particularly Black Triangle, have spent two years campaigning for wider awareness of regulation 35, which they believe can save lives if used more often. It has been campaigning to force the British Medical Association (BMA) to tell every GP about the regulation, which the BMA will finally agree to do the following spring. Litchfield concludes that regulation 35 appears to be 'the main driver' for a sharp rise in the proportion of new claimants being placed in the support group and suggests these positive developments should be reversed. Campaigners have been fending off attempts to remove this safety net since Treasury officials first raised concerns about it in September 1994.

Litchfield briefly mentions the report into the death of Ms DE but says only that it highlighted 'the issue of correctly identifying individuals at risk of self-harm and suicide'. There is no mention of peer reviews or of any prevention of future deaths reports.

17
The Death of Faiza Ahmed

> People understand I jus wanna lucky break after all I work as hard as u, n even harder dan u so cum on yall give gal dem a chance cos it seemz 2 me if I dnt get dat 1 chance I ma break down n start drinkin heavy, takin drugz maybe even go out n get locked [imprisoned] but I dnt wanna b a failure all my life I wanna make mum happy n proud cos everything I do is 4 her because if it weren't 4 my mum den I would b in a coffin, in a graveyard facin my judgementz in da hereafter.

There is a sapphire blue grill across the entrance to Sailors Palace, an intercom, and two steps down to the pavement. Faiza turns right from the block of flats where she lives in Limehouse, east London, and walks along the six-lane West India Dock Road, clogged with traffic, a typical east London mix of takeaways and blocks of flats, four and five storeys high. Looming in the distance is Canary Wharf. Most striking among the skyscrapers ahead of her is the giant logo marking out the HSBC headquarters.

A minute or so's walk and she turns right towards Westferry DLR. The Docklands Light Railway crosses above the street and she walks alongside and beneath it before turning sharply right. Ignoring the sign reminding her to 'please touch in and out', she mounts the 40 or so steps to the eastbound platform. It is 6.09pm on 7 November 2014.

* * *

Faiza was born in Somalia but moves to London with her family as a toddler. She has six sisters but is closest to her brother Mo, who is a year older. The two of them are different to their siblings, less inclined to stick to the rules, more willing to challenge authority. Mo says they were 'thick as thieves', always covering each other's backs. He says his sister was misunderstood, often angry and resisting rules and those in charge, but he believes she was 'over-disciplined'. Her teachers were too quick to give up on her, did too little to understand the anger. There are school expulsions, fights with local children, arguments at home, arrests for shoplifting.

At 14 comes an incident that leaves her permanently scarred. She is arrested for a minor offence and held at the local police station. Her father is on the way to collect her when he is hit by a car. He dies several days later. For the rest of her life, as her family would learn only later, she will blame herself for his death.

She leaves school with few qualifications. There is intermittent employment, some training, periods of unemployment. She serves a couple of months in prison when she is 20 for assaulting a police officer. Her criminal record holds her back. She loves music and poetry, but struggles to find a way forward. That is until 2012.

Along with many other young people from disadvantaged backgrounds, the organisers of London 2012 – the London Olympic and Paralympic Games – give her a chance. She secures a temporary job as a team leader in nearby Stratford, and just for a few months in that one summer when nearly anything seems possible in the capital, she flourishes. Mo remembers her being 'so happy'. It would have been easy for the organisers to give her a token job, but she is a team leader with real responsibility. And for a few months, she has an opportunity to demonstrate her potential.

'I'd never seen her so committed,' Mo would say later. 'She was working long hours at the Olympic Village. She was there until late, she was leaving early, she was exhausted every single day. I'd never seen her like that, with that kind of passion, she had such a spring in her step. It was unreal.'

But soon London 2012 is over, and Faiza is back signing on at Poplar jobcentre, in Dod Street, just a few minutes' walk from her flat. The Dod Street jobcentre has closed now, and is scheduled for demolition, to be replaced with a block of flats. But in the spring of 2022, it is still possible to peer through the windows and see a grim space, a partly laminated floor and grey carpet squares, mostly open-plan, low-ceilinged, with little natural light.

Mo remembers the Dod Street jobcentre as a 'toxic' place – he experienced it himself briefly after leaving school. 'The people who worked there looked at you as if you were the lowest of the low,' he told me. 'Everything was a threat. If you were a couple of minutes late, you were told you'd be sanctioned next time.'

Mo calls his sister Sophie, a name she came up with because of a teacher's inability to pronounce her name. She needs to be at the jobcentre early because they have threatened her with a sanction for being late. There is, he says, a 'sense of edge' about her dealings with the jobcentre. She is being told she hasn't carried out enough job searches, and has to apply for jobs she has no interest in. She develops an interest in working with children, but it is difficult with her criminal record.

'It was a horrible, horrible place for her,' says Mo. 'Whenever we saw her, she was absolutely broken from it. She was scared, worried and upset. She was a strong, independent person but she knew that if she was sanctioned, she would have nothing. As much as we were there to help her, both financially and emotionally, she wanted to do things for herself, so she was too proud to ask for anything.' The jobcentre never really believed her when she said she had depression.

Mo had his own brushes with the law as a teenager. He then joins the Parachute Regiment and the experience has a profound impact. 'You were trained to be a killer,' he will say later. 'I also started drinking. To fit in, you really had to drink.' The combination of drinking and aggression is a toxic mix. One night, after he and his colleagues represent the regiment by working as stewards at a Southend football match, they head out on the town. Later, Mo is waiting for a cab, and another man tries to jump the queue, possibly not realising Mo is ahead of him. 'I head-butted him and hit him a couple of times and he fell onto the floor.'

Mo, who is 22, is given six months for actual bodily harm, partly because of a juvenile record of theft and assault. He serves a month at Belmarsh and another month at Elmley on the Isle of Sheppey.

It is a life-changing experience. 'I felt fearful for my life,' he says, 'depressed, suicidal thoughts.'

It is Faiza who 'stepped up'. She visits Mo with their mum, and writes him letters, encouraging him, joking, telling her brother she believes in him. In one letter, she tells him to 'stay out of trouble', 'keep busy', not to give up hope. She tells her brother how much he is loved, and how his mother – who Faiza adores – is proud of 'who u were, are + who u'll becum inshallah!'

In another, she responds to one of Mo's letters, in which he reveals his depression, and says the family feel 'helpless' they can't be there by his side to support him.

The letters his 'stubborn' and 'strong-willed' sister writes to him give him the strength he needs to survive prison and turn his life around. Several years later, he joins the fire service, and he still serves today as an officer with London Fire Brigade. 'No-one else wrote to me,' he said later. 'She did what she had done all my life. She really stepped up and showed how much she cared. She gave me immense courage and that has stuck with me my entire life. If she hadn't stuck with me then, who knows?'

Mo and his sister remained close, and he would usually see her at least once a week. But in the days leading up to 7 November he is recovering from an accident. He has been temporarily based in Brighton and had fallen through a ceiling while attending a fire. His wrist is pinned. Faiza winds him up about the accident when they talk on the phone. Only later does he discover she had been struggling, drinking heavily and taking soft drugs, and how traumatic the last few days had been.

Faiza was diagnosed with a personality disorder in 2010. She was sectioned under the Mental Health Act in 2011, attempted suicide in 2013, and in 2014 disclosed further suicidal thoughts to her GP. In the late summer, she discloses that she is drinking heavily and not eating properly, although she mentions a supportive partner.

On the evening of Thursday 6 November, her partner and a friend have been drinking until the early hours at Faiza's flat. Her partner leaves for work, but the friend stays in the flat. Faiza goes to bed.

An inquest will hear how Faiza turns up later at the door of a downstairs neighbour, in a state of extreme distress, saying the friend has tried to rape her, and asking the woman to call the police.

A police review will describe how officers found Faiza outside her flat with blood on her clothes. She tells them she has been drinking through the night but refuses to let them take the clothing and bedding for examination. They try to persuade her not to return to her flat as it is a potential crime scene.

The neighbour later expresses surprise at the intrusiveness of the questioning by a male police officer about a sexual assault in a communal part of the building. She tells the inquest the questioning was matter-of-fact, and she 'thought they would be much softer'. She says this appears to have increased Faiza's hostility towards the officers.

By now there are four officers at the scene, with two of them – including a female officer – interviewing the friend upstairs, and two male officers with Faiza.

They establish some basic facts, and arrest her friend. But the more the male officers probe Faiza, the more hostile she becomes, eventually telling them: 'You lot don't want to know. You are heavyweight bullies. He won't go to prison. Fuck off. I hope *you* get raped. You can't do anything.'

Faiza eventually returns to her flat. By now, the police have checked their records, which describe Faiza as capable of being 'volatile and violent' when drunk and state that she assaulted officers in her flat five months earlier while they were checking on her welfare. A senior officer tells a female specialist sexual offences officer who is on the way to Faiza's flat (and had forgotten her personal protective equipment) to return to the station. A detective sergeant arranges for the officer and a colleague to return the following day.

What happens over the following 24 hours is unclear, although a post-mortem will suggest Faiza continued drinking. At about 2pm, Faiza attends Poplar jobcentre. She had been due to see her work coach three days earlier but phoned in sick. She is asked to fill in a JSA28 form to explain her illness. She fills in the form and, the work coach says later – a claim Mo has always distrusted – that she leaves while he is reading it. Asked to provide 'brief details of your sickness', she has written: 'I was busy trying to kill myself, drinking non-stop.'

The work coach insists later that she seemed calm and not upset and not about to take her own life. He cannot explain why he did not call the emergency services, and insists Faiza filled in the form to show she was now 'better'.

He discusses the form with his manager, and they say they follow DWP's 'six-point plan' framework, designed for when claimants say they intend to self-harm or take their own lives. Five days later, the jobcentre contacts the community mental health team to tell them about Faiza's statement.

DWP will later say the work coach 'made a judgement that there was no immediate risk to her safety'. That judgement is fatally flawed.

Faiza returns to her flat and continues drinking. At 4.05pm, she calls 999. The inquest will hear a transcript of that call. Faiza tells the operator she is trying to slit her wrist and needs help. She says she is in her flat with a piece of glass.

She tells the operator: 'I'm very scared. I had too much to drink, and I'm sorry, like. I don't want to live no more. I just want to die. There's nothing to live for. There's no one with me. I just want to die. I just want to die.' She then tells the operator she doesn't want an ambulance and hangs up.

But despite the clarity of her call, paramedics are only told that she has been 'trying to slit her wrists' and there was a 'suicide attempt' and she is 'armed with a weapon – glass'. But they are not told she wants to die. Because of the reference to a 'weapon', London Ambulance Service calls the police.

Neither the paramedics nor the police officers are aware of her history of mental distress and suicide attempts, that she has previously been sectioned, or that she reported an attempted rape the previous day. Crucially, the police arrive before the ambulance.

On arrival, one of the two male police officers knocks on her door, and Faiza asks who it is.

One of the officers says: 'It's the police. Can you open the door please?'

'Everything is fine,' she replies. 'There is no crime here.'

'Can you open the door, as I don't want to force it open? We just need to speak with you, that's all.'

Faiza opens the door, and she says: 'I don't need you lot. You can fuck off.'

When the officer explains they have been asked to attend by the ambulance service, because of someone threatening to harm themselves with a piece of glass, she says: 'Well it's not me. I don't need you lot here. I never asked you to come so can you please fuck off.'

'Have you hurt yourself with some glass?'

'No,' she says.

'What's your name?' he asks.

'You don't need to know my name, it's all on your systems,' says Faiza.

'Have you called for an ambulance?'

'No, I don't need an ambulance and I don't know why you are here.'

'Could anybody else have called an ambulance for you? Have you phoned a friend or anybody to say you were going to hurt yourself with some glass?'

'No,' she says. 'Look, I never called you lot, please fuck off.'

The paramedics soon arrive and take over. It is only now that two officers from the sexual offences unit arrive. They appear to have waited outside the flat for five minutes, and receive a briefing from a colleague about what they have deduced about Faiza's 'state of mind and volatility'. The paramedics tell them there are no immediate welfare concerns.

The two specialist officers leave without talking to Faiza. They fail to tell the paramedics about the rape allegation, and, in the words of the coroner, this information is 'not adequately conveyed to the police response team'. The paramedics will later say they would have behaved differently if they had known about the rape allegation. The police officers and the paramedics have left the flat by 5.30pm, having decided Faiza is not at immediate risk of harming herself.

At some point between 5.30pm and 6pm, Faiza writes the following note:

This is to ~~everyone I love~~ my family, including you wifey [Faiza's nickname for her boyfriend]. I have had enough. I just want to sleep forever! Please forgive me for exiting the world the way I did. Thankyou wife for loving me! Mum I'm sorry. The pain of feelin alone got too much!

She leaves the flat and heads towards Westferry DLR station.

'She was my favourite sister,' says Mo, years later, 'which the rest of my sisters don't like … She would always be willing to try to help anyone. I know it's a cliché, but she would give anyone her last five pounds. She was such a wonderful, generous person.'

He speaks of Faiza's connection with his daughter, who adored her aunt and was devastated when she died. And he is filled with regret that his son, born in 2019, will never meet his aunt, although he promises he will tell him one day what a wonderful, strong person she was. 'Even now,' he says, 'I take a lot of strength from my sister when I am down or upset, when people are against me, when my back is against the wall. I think, "What would Sophie do? She wouldn't just take it."'

Mo hears about his beloved sister's death via a WhatsApp message. He is recuperating at his girlfriend's house and had turned his phone off overnight. He wakes to a message from one of his sisters to say the police were knocking on the door at 3am and Faiza has taken her own life. 'I just completely broke down and cried non-stop,' says Mo.

A few days later, someone from Poplar jobcentre calls the devastated family. They are worried about Faiza and are trying to contact her. One of her sisters tells the jobcentre officer that Faiza 'is not with us anymore', she has taken her own life.

When Mo hears about the call, he becomes suspicious. He believes someone looked at the paperwork and panicked. He hopes Faiza's suicide was because she couldn't cope with her depression, but he wants to be sure nothing triggered her decision to take her own life.

Mo starts to piece together the last couple of days of Faiza's life. Years of *Newsnight* and Radio 4 reassure him that if he keeps asking questions, the answers will come. He puts in a subject access request to DWP for any information they have about Faiza. 'It was the suspicions I had from all the years leading up to this, how they treated her,' Mo tells me. 'She'd been sanctioned at least once within the last 18 months, and I think she'd been threatened on a number of occasions. When you sanction someone, you know that they're not going to have any money or any food. How is that humane in any way? That's why I was always suspicious, because I felt that an organisation that treats someone like that, it is possible they could have done any number of things that sent her over the edge.'

A helpful British Transport Police officer tells the family there was police contact in the days before Faiza's death. 'I start going down to the police station, to the jobcentre. The defensiveness of both of them was so much that we knew something was up,' says Mo. He starts to realise the horror of Faiza's last couple of days, and that the agencies that were supposed to be there to help had failed her.

'When you create what is a hostile environment at the very top, the people on the ground are not going to be any different. Austerity and hostility are completely bound up with each other. And you can't take the race element out of it. Poverty disproportionately impacts people from BME backgrounds. And it's not the people in the jobcentre being directly racist, because many of them are BME people, it's the policy which is at the heart of it.'

It also helps explain the behaviour of the police and ambulance service, he says. 'There is the casual racism of a young black woman being emotional and upset and that being seen as aggressive and confrontational.'

He is supported by campaign group Women Against Rape, help which Mo says was crucial in his fight for justice. With this help, he successfully takes the coroner to the high court to ensure there is an Article 2 inquest, to examine if the state has failed in its obligation to protect Faiza's right to life.

Despite Mo's fears that the inquest will be a cover-up, it lasts eight days and is thorough, with a jury, and there is evidence from police, paramedics, and the work coach who spoke to Faiza on the day she died, who insists she left while he was reading the form in which she said she was 'busy trying to kill myself'.

Under the six-point plan, staff should summon emergency help if a claimant declares an attempt to kill themselves and is 'distressed, at serious risk or in immediate danger'. Instead, the inquest hears, the jobcentre did not contact the community mental health team for five days. The work coach cannot explain why Faiza's statement did not prompt a call to the police.

The inquest jury returns a narrative verdict, concluding that the police, ambulance service, and jobcentre each contributed to Faiza's suicide. It describes the 'historical and continuing lack of rapport' between Faiza and the police, which contributed to her not receiving the support she needed, the ambulance crew that was 'insufficiently informed', and how the jobcentre missed an 'opportunity to alert the relevant authorities'. The coroner, Mary Hassell, says the failings are so serious she will write a prevention of future deaths (PFD) report, to the Metropolitan police, London Ambulance Service, and DWP.[1]

Mo still hopes another family will not have to experience what his have been through. 'That would give me a lot of happiness and peace, because it would mean that Faiza's death wasn't for nothing.' But he knows the deaths have kept happening. 'What has changed?' he says. 'Can I see what happened to my sister happening today? A hundred per cent yes.'

I only learn of her death in the summer of 2020, after another freedom of information request. At the time of the inquest, in February 2016, I had missed the lengthy, powerful article about Faiza's death written by *The Guardian*'s Simon Hattenstone.[2]

The freedom of information request reveals DWP's response to Mary Hassell's PFD report, which had not previously been published due, says the Judicial Office, to an 'administrative oversight'. It shows DWP – again – has dismissed a coroner's call to take action to make its procedures safer.

In its response, DWP says: 'In this case, based on the information he had, the Work Coach made a judgement that there was no immediate risk to her safety.' DWP claims its processes 'were followed both diligently and correctly', and staff 'took the necessary steps to invoke the agreed processes that would manage the risk appropriately'. The department adds: 'It is not our view that any opportunity to engage with any other organisations was missed.'

It says the only action it will take will be to issue a reminder to all DWP staff about its existing guidance on suicidal ideation, the same guidance which failed Faiza Ahmed. Yet again, DWP's response to a death is defensive, stubborn, and complacent.

PART IV

2014–22
Cover-up, Investigations, and the Truth about DWP

18

Michael O'Sullivan, and the Prevention of Future Deaths

In the autumn of 2015, while still mired in the legal battle with DWP over the unpublished peer reviews, I start to think again about the deaths, and where official records might be held. There seems no way to find out how often DWP is being asked to give evidence to inquests, but the Coroners' Society – which represents coroners in England and Wales – tells me about prevention of future deaths (PFD) reports. Although they will only cover a minority of deaths linked to the department, they should bring to light some of the worst cases. PFD reports from July 2013 onwards are held publicly, online, by the Ministry of Justice. I start searching the archives. Just one report catches my eye. It mentions DWP and the suicide of 60-year-old Michael O'Sullivan.[1]

Michael had been claiming incapacity benefit since 2000, following a breakdown, due to depression, social anxiety, agoraphobia, and general anxiety disorder that had gradually intensified since he moved to London from County Kerry in rural Ireland at the age of 19. He was the youngest of five children and had been a happy and much-loved child.

He was one of hundreds of thousands of former claimants of incapacity benefit, disability-based income support, and severe disablement allowance who were assessed for the new ESA as part of the 'migration process' launched by Grayling and Duncan Smith in 2011. Michael was told in March 2012 that he would be reassessed. In the following months, his family noticed his low moods, that he was constantly worried, and stopped watching television and listening to the radio. He was frightened by the idea of returning to work, and losing his benefits and independence.

He was assessed in August by a young physiotherapist, an assessment that lasted just twelve minutes and left him 'humiliated, mortified, and feeling like a criminal', reducing him to tears when he described the experience to his daughter Anne-Marie. He was declared fit for work, and although he asked DWP to reconsider, his appeal was rejected. He began experiencing severe anxiety and panic attacks.

He was told to attend a two-week training course – to qualify for the card necessary to work on a building site – at a college in Tottenham. Surrounded by 70 other far younger students, he was constantly mocked and harassed. At the end of the first week, he could not face returning, and tried to end his own life. He was deemed unfit for work for six months by his GP but was called for another WCA just four months later.

This time, he was assessed at Atos's Marylebone assessment centre by Dr Fathy Awad Sherif, a former orthopaedic surgeon who had worked for the company for 15 years. At the inquest into Michael's death, Dr Sherif claimed he had not asked Michael if he had suicidal thoughts because he 'looked OK'. He wrote in three places that Michael had 'no ideas of self-harm', even though he had failed to ask him and despite Michael making it clear on his pre-assessment form that he had suicidal thoughts. Dr Sherif said claimants sometimes fake their symptoms, and he had not wanted to 'place' the idea of suicide in Michael's head. He admitted Michael looked 'a bit stressed' but insisted this was perfectly normal for people who claimed they were depressed, and was just a sign they were worried about losing their benefits.

Dr Sherif failed to seek evidence from any of Michael's doctors, telling him the DWP decision-maker would look at that information instead. But the DWP decision-maker did not request any reports or letters from Michael's GP (who had concluded he was not well enough to work), his psychiatrist (who had diagnosed him with recurrent depression and panic disorder with agoraphobia), or his clinical psychologist (who had assessed him as 'very anxious and showing signs of clinical depression').

Dr Sherif took just 21 minutes to assess Michael, and only another eleven minutes to complete the paperwork. He concluded that Michael was 'at no significant risk by working' and found him fit for work.

Michael was placed on jobseeker's allowance. He applied for countless jobs, and was scrupulous in meeting the strict terms of his jobseeker's agreement. Just one employer replied. He was eventually told to attend a four-week job placement as a labourer on a demolition site and had to buy his own safety hat, steel-capped boots and high-vis jacket. In the week leading up to the placement, he looked withdrawn, and struggled to eat or sleep properly. After washing and ironing five shirts for the week ahead, he took his own life on Monday 23 September 2013.

There were 14 missed calls on his phone from the agency that placed him on the job. Anne-Marie says the family will never know if his life had ended by the time they began hounding him, or if the pressure of those calls triggered his decision to take his own life.

* * *

The coroner's office had been told about the links between his suicide and DWP's actions by Anne-Marie, who would spend the next decade searching for justice, and the truth about her father's death. Her serious concerns led to the inquest being adjourned, allowing an in-depth investigation.

Mary Hassell, the senior coroner for inner north London, ensured that Michael's GP, psychiatrist, and psychologist gave evidence at the inquest. She also ordered Dr Sherif to give evidence but he failed to turn up – claiming he had forgotten – and had to be summonsed to appear.

At the end of the inquest, in January 2014, Hassell – who had also led the Faiza Ahmed inquest – ruled that the 'trigger' for Michael's suicide was being found fit for work. 'The anxiety and depression were long term problems,' she wrote, 'but the intense anxiety that triggered his suicide was caused by his recent assessment by the Department for Work and Pensions (benefits agency) as being fit for work, and his view of the likely consequences of that.' Just as Tom Osborne had done four years earlier, Hassell concluded there was 'a risk that future deaths will occur unless action is taken', and she sent her report to DWP.

I publish an article about Hassell's report, on 18 September 2015, although I don't use Michael's name as I have yet to track down the family.[2]

In its response to Mary Hassell's PFD report, DWP claimed it had a 'clear policy' that further medical evidence should be requested in cases 'where claimants report suicidal ideation in their claim forms', which 'regrettably was not followed in this instance'. It planned to remind staff. But it also said it was 'important to retain a balance between the added value of further evidence in any claim for ESA and time demands on GPs and other healthcare professionals'. It concluded: 'We have noted the issues in this case and will continue to monitor our policies around assessment of people with mental health problems while we await the outcome of related litigation.'

This 'related litigation' was the further medical evidence court case that was still crawling its way through the legal system, plagued by DWP delays and obstruction. Earlier in 2015, the upper tribunal administrative appeals chamber had dismissed the two claimants' cases,[3] saying they had not proved they themselves had faced discrimination. But the court still concluded that the WCA discriminated against some disabled people. It also criticised the 'frustrating' responses of Iain Duncan Smith and DWP's delay in piloting improvements to the further medical evidence process.

Anne-Marie – who will submit written evidence about her father's case to the UN inquiry – tells me DWP's failings had been 'catastrophic' and had a 'devastating' impact on the family. 'As far as we can see, they have done nothing to change the system since he died,' she says. 'We will never recover from our loss. It will haunt us for the rest of our lives because it should and could have been avoided. Now we just hope his life will prove not to have been lost in vain.'

Just a week after I break the Michael O'Sullivan story, DWP orders Maximus to send a memo to all staff engaged in 'filework' – preparing files for claimants ahead of their assessment. The memo will only be revealed twelve months later by the Benefits and Work website, following a freedom of information battle with DWP.[4] DWP demands 'written confirmation' from each staff member that they have read the memo.

It refers to two 'historical cases', one of them Michael O'Sullivan's, where DWP has been 'challenged' over a decision not to request further medical evidence ahead of an assessment. In both cases 'there has ultimately been a tragic outcome'. The memo reminds staff that the guidance – since December 2010 – states that, where there is reference to a previous suicide attempt, suicidal ideation or self-harm on the ESA questionnaire, the healthcare professional must request further medical evidence. It adds: 'If you follow the guidance then we can defend you should a tragic incident occur. If you do not follow the guidance we cannot. I am sure most people's reaction will be that you all already do this. Unfortunately we have clear evidence where it has not occurred.'

DWP is not suggesting new measures to make the WCA system safer or to ensure further medical evidence is requested in more cases, but is simply restating existing guidance. This refusal to make the system safer means claimants will continue to die unnecessary deaths.

Following the DNS stories on Michael O'Sullivan, and a report by *ITV News*, Michael's case is mentioned in consecutive weeks at prime minister's questions by the SNP's Angus Robertson.

David Cameron says it would not be appropriate to 'discuss the specifics of the cases' although suicide is 'always a tragic and complex issue'. He claims any peer review of Michael's death cannot be published 'because it has personal and medical data in it which would not be appropriate for publication'.[5]

Meanwhile, Iain Duncan Smith is paying no attention to the lethal impact of his policies, telling the Conservative conference in Manchester: 'The evidence of our reforms is that people respond to incentives. We know that. We know that in our hearts. With our help, I say to them, you will work your way out of poverty. That is the pledge we make to those who need our support.'[6] Just a day earlier, chancellor George Osborne had made repeated references to the need to deliver 'lower welfare'.

Meanwhile, disabled activists and allies are protesting outside the conference, led by Disabled People Against Cuts (DPAC), with some of the angriest scenes seen under successive Conservative-led governments. The protesters include relatives of two disabled people whose deaths have been linked to DWP reforms.

Nichole Drury tells me how her mother's out-of-work benefits were removed because she had twice been too unwell to attend a work capability assessment. Her mother, Moira, spent the last six months of her life fighting DWP over its decision. She told her daughter, before she died, that the stress of this battle had contributed to her deteriorating health. Nichole had travelled to Manchester because, she says, 'the system is cruel and it is unfair and it seems like the weakest and most vulnerable are being targeted by the cuts. People like my mum don't fight back because they can't.'

Natalie Jeffers also joins disabled activists outside the conference. Her brother Luke Alexander Loy, who had schizophrenia, had been claiming incapacity benefit for more than 20 years and had been in a 'very good rhythm', taking five walks a day, working on art projects as therapy, and shopping for his elderly neighbour. But he was caught up in the reassessment process. He was found fit for work, despite his doctor explaining he was not well enough for a job. He had apparently been sanctioned for failing to attend meetings and not actively looking for work, and he fell deep into debt, becoming withdrawn and scared. After his father discovered what had happened, he helped his son appeal and eventually DWP reinstated his benefits. By then the damage had been done. His family had become concerned about his welfare, and police officers broke into his house and found him dead on his bedroom floor. An inquest reached an open verdict.

Natalie tells me: 'We can't prove the cause of my brother's death, but we know that the only seismic shift in his life that shocked his stability and impacted a decline in his mental health was this WCA decision.' She is appalled by the 'vicious' and 'despicable' conference speech given by Iain Duncan Smith, which appears aimed at tarring disabled people as 'scroungers'. Instead of creating compassion, she says, the government was creating a culture of fear.

Soon afterwards, I receive a freedom of information response from the Ministry of Justice. I had asked how to find the PFD reports that pre-dated July 2013, and for copies of any such reports sent to DWP. I am told the Ministry of Justice publishes six-monthly summaries, but coroners only began sending copies of their PFD reports to central government in July 2008. It means it is impossible to know whether any coroners drew links between DWP (or DSS) and the deaths of claimants before 2008.

The Ministry of Justice provides links to summaries from 2008 to 2013 and attaches three PFD reports. One is dated March 2010. It is Tom Osborne's report, sent to DWP following the Stephen Carré inquest. I read Osborne's conclusions about the WCA being a trigger for Stephen's suicide, and the failure to seek further medical evidence. The scale of DWP's deceit, negligence, and recklessness had suddenly become clear.

Stephen's sister Sarah is horrified when I tell her of DWP's failures. 'I knew that governments didn't really care about the lives of ordinary people, but this took it to the next level,' she tells me, years later. 'To hear that the coroner had contacted the government, warning of the risk to life, and that the government had disregarded the warning, causing further deaths, was chilling. This felt like a deliberate act intended to save money by killing claimants.

'For one claimant to be treated so dishonestly could be blamed on one employee of the system, with others trying to cover up the mess. But to hear about others showed that this "was" the system, that the corporate policy was to find as many claimants "fit for work" as possible, no matter the impact on the individuals, or the truth. I hadn't realised how much of what I considered to be public sector work was being contracted out to private companies, whose whole reason for being was to make as much profit as possible, by whatever means necessary. This was capitalism at its worst.'

Sarah still struggles to understand the morality of those involved, and not just the senior civil servants, but those making the day-to-day decisions. 'I didn't – and don't – understand how they could go home to their families, knowing that they've behaved like this. And each new death that I hear about reinforces all of these feelings.'

But there is even more to this story. Sarah Carré herself had been diagnosed with a mental health condition in her early 20s, and was hospitalised in her late 20s. 'The benefits system back then wasn't pleasant,' she says, 'but did allow me the time to recover without too much pressure. I had another bad episode about five years later, and recovered without pressure.'

Then, in 2013, she made what she describes as a serious suicide attempt. It was more than a year before she could return to work, although she didn't claim benefits during this period. She was passionate about her work, and highly motivated to recover. But in 2018, she again became very ill, and had to start claiming benefits. 'The change since the last time was horrendous,' she says. 'From day one, I could tell that it was designed to be as humiliating as possible. I was quite lucky with my jobcentre adviser, as she had experienced mental health issues herself in the past, but even she wasn't able to protect me from the worst of the system.'

She was eventually placed on ESA, and that, she says, 'is when the real nightmare started'. 'I was very poorly. Probably as bad as I could get without making another suicide attempt. I still needed to fill the forms in, but all of the organisations supposedly set up to help with the form-filling were too busy to help me before the deadline, so I just had to manage.'

She included evidence from her medical records, including details of her hospitalisations, letters from the hospital, and her suicide attempt. 'I was worried about dealing with the DWP after what had happened to Stephen, so when I got the letter telling me that I had to go for a work capability assessment I went into a tailspin. Everyone who interacted with me, or even looked at me, could tell that there was something seriously wrong.' A friend insisted on accompanying her to the assessment, so she could take notes.

When they arrived, she was told she could not be accompanied, but she could have the assessment recorded. They had no recording equipment available, so she was sent another appointment. At the next appointment, she was told again that there was no equipment available.

She finally had the assessment and cried through the interview. The questions were focused on her physical health, with few about her mental distress. She was found fit for work. 'The justification for that bore no resemblance to any of the information on the form, to any of the medical records that I had sent, and told me that I had been calm, responsive, and capable during my assessment,' she says. 'I couldn't believe that this was actually happening. After all of these years since Stephen's death they were still ignoring evidence, still lying about the assessment, and still treating people with high risks of suicide in this way.

'It took every ounce of my determination not to give up there and then. I don't think that it was a desire to live – once I'd made that serious suicide attempt, I no longer feared dying – but was more because I didn't want the DWP to reduce their benefits payout by killing me. I wrote to them, reminding them of my previous attempt, and pointing out that Stephen had been the first. Did they want it in the media that two people from the same family had died as a direct result of their policies?' DWP phoned Sarah on the day they received the letter, telling her they had overturned their original decision.

A few months later, her employer granted her ill-health retirement. 'I don't have a big pension,' she says, 'just enough to keep me out of the DWP clutches. But hearing that set me on the path of recovery.' Sarah says she will never be well enough to work full time, but she has built a life for herself that allows her to stay as well as possible. 'I am very happy,' she tells me. 'I would not be able to feel like this if I knew that I would have to tackle the DWP regularly, and I don't think that I would have survived another episode with them.

'What makes me really sad is that none of it was necessary. Not what happened to Stephen, not what happened to any of the other people who have died, and not what happened to me. Some people aren't fit for work. Some people will never be fit for work. But if the DWP worked in conjunction with doctors, hospitals, and claimants themselves, they would get better outcomes for all concerned. Instead, they declare war on the most vulnerable in our society.'

So why did the prevention of future deaths report written by the coroner at the inquest into Stephen Carré's death prove to be so important? There are three key reasons.

It showed that DWP and its ministers and senior civil servants were warned by a coroner about the fatal risks and flaws inherent in the work capability assessment, and that they needed to make significant changes to the process to prevent further deaths. The Michael O'Sullivan PFD report showed that they refused to do anything except make minor changes to their Atos filework guidance in December 2010. Michael's deaths, and so many others, only happened because of that failure.

Secondly, employment minister Chris Grayling and work and pensions secretary Iain Duncan Smith decided in the summer of 2010 that Labour's work capability assessment could be rolled out the following spring to people who had been claiming long-term incapacity benefit. This was despite being shown the Stephen Carré PFD report and being told it was too soon for the rollout by Professor Malcolm Harrington, their own independent reviewer. They knew the risks, and yet they went ahead and applied the assessment to hundreds of thousands of people, many with long-term mental distress.

Perhaps most disturbing, I soon discover that ministers failed to share the Stephen Carré PFD report with Professor Harrington, who told me:

> I cannot recall the report. Nobody brought it to my attention that I can remember. If I had known about that coroner's report, I would have said that this was something else we need to look at. I am a doctor, I know about coroner's reports. Coroner's reports are something that you don't ignore.

He says the need to secure further medical evidence was a consistent concern during the three reviews he carried out – in 2010, 2011, and 2012 – and he made it clear in his third review that decision-makers should 'actively' consider seeking further medical evidence. If he had been shown the coroner's letter, he says, it would almost certainly have led to him making recommendations far earlier about the need to seek further medical evidence. He says this is particularly important for claimants with mental distress, like Stephen Carré.

'Of course!' he tells me. 'They weren't picking up this additional information that should have been right up front. It would have brought forward the best evidence.' Asked how he felt about Grayling's failure to pass on this information to him, he says: 'No comment.'

In February 2016, following months of DNS reports, DWP suddenly uncovers the response that should have been sent to Tom Osborne in the summer of 2010. It is predictably defensive. DWP says it 'remains unclear to us how further medical evidence would have changed the outcome', and that the inquest evidence given by Stephen's psychiatrist indicated that 'at no time did any of his team report any concerns that he was at serious risk of taking his own life'. DWP insists Stephen was fit for work at the time he was assessed. It offers a detailed defence of the WCA and ends by stating: 'I regret the unfortunate circumstances surrounding the death of Mr Carré but I hope this reply will re-assure you that in this case the DWP acted responsibly and appropriately.'

Years later, in 2022, I try to secure the transcript of Stephen's inquest. I am told by Bedfordshire and Luton Coroner's Service that a recording is no longer available, and neither is the transcript. Tom Osborne's notes are also missing from the archive file. Osborne's new office, in Milton Keynes, tells me

> his usual practice would be for any documents obtained by him, such as a transcript of a hearing, to be filed with the inquest record. I understand that a thorough search has taken place and this has not been found and I can appreciate the frustration this causes but I can confirm that Mr Osborne does not personally hold any records with regard to this matter.

Somehow, in the intervening years, both the transcript and the recording of the Stephen Carré inquest have vanished.

19

Iain Duncan Smith, the UN, and 590 Suicides

Soon after the discovery of the Stephen Carré PFD report comes the research evidence disabled activists have been seeking for years. Public health experts from the Universities of Liverpool and Oxford show that for every 10,000 incapacity benefit claimants who were reassessed through the WCA in England between 2010 and 2013, there were an additional six suicides, 2,700 cases of self-reported mental health problems, and an increase of more than 7,000 in the number of anti-depressants prescribed.[1] The most significant increases took place in the most deprived areas. Across England, the reassessment process from 2010 to 2013 was 'associated with' an extra 590 suicides.

The idea for the research had come from disabled activists including Rick Burgess, who co-founded the grassroots campaign group New Approach and had been involved with the WOW (War on Welfare) campaign. The WOW campaign had led to a Commons debate that called on the government to assess the cumulative impact of all its welfare cuts on disabled people.

Burgess wanted 'recognised and respected epidemiologists' to carry out 'an academically-rigorous study' into the number of deaths caused by the WCA. Together with three other campaigners – artist-activist Liz Crow and New Approach co-founder Jane Bence and welfare rights expert Nick Dilworth (who will work for years with the O'Sullivan family on their quest for justice) – Burgess began discussing the idea with David Stuckler, professor of political economy and sociology at Oxford.

They hoped the research would be completed in time for the 2015 general election, but that was not to be, and the Conservative Party won a slim overall majority, with a manifesto promising to cut social security spending by a further £12 billion a year. When Stuckler and his colleagues publish their findings in November 2015, Burgess feels 'grimly vindicated'.

DWP describes the findings as 'wholly misleading' and says 'the authors themselves caution that no conclusions can be drawn about cause and effect'. DWP also points to the five independent reviews of the WCA and the 'significant improvements to the process' since 2010.

Ben Barr, the study's lead author and a senior clinical lecturer in applied public health research at the University of Liverpool, says none of the other factors the researchers had considered as possible causes could explain the rise in suicides. The increases only happened among age groups most affected by the WCA, while the rise in mental distress 'tended to occur shortly after the increase in people undergoing the WCA in each area'.

'Unfortunately, the DWP implemented the policy without a controlled trial or any plans to evaluate its impact on mental health,' he says. 'Given that data is not currently available on the specific individuals who underwent the WCA and there is no trial evidence, the next best approach to investigate the potential effects on mental health is the one we applied in our study, using appropriate statistical methods to control for alternative explanations for these trends.'

Another academic, Ben Baumberg Geiger, will say later that the reaction to the study within DWP was quite different to its public response. He had been on secondment to DWP at the time and told the Deaths by Welfare podcast in 2023[2] that people within the department were reading and 'paying attention' to the findings. He was asked to brief various teams about its contents.

The previous month, the new government's Welfare Reform and Work Bill had had its first reading. The bill will remove the extra payment given to claimants in the ESA work-related activity group, removing nearly £30 per week from hundreds of thousands of disabled people on out-of-work benefits, driving them further into poverty. The legislation will be passed by parliament in March 2016.[3]

Any doubt that DWP is still trying to make the assessment process steadily more violent is dispelled in December 2015. It issues updated guidance to Maximus, the contractor that has taken over the WCA contract from Atos.[4]

The new guidance makes it harder for claimants at significant risk of harm because of their mental health to avoid work-related activity, following the recommendation made by Paul Litchfield in his final review of the WCA twelve months earlier.

The previous version of DWP's WCA handbook stated that if a claimant was currently sectioned, had active thoughts of suicide, or had a documented episode of self-harm requiring medical attention in the last twelve months, it should be seen as a 'definitive' 'substantial risk' that meant they should be placed in the ESA support group. But the new guidance tells assessors that such indicators 'might' give rise to a substantial risk in 'exceptional circumstances' and that they should weigh 'the benefits of employment … against any potential risk'.

Following these changes, the proportion of ESA claimants placed in the support group plunges by two-fifths in three months, while the proportion found fit for work rises from 35 to 49 per cent and those told to carry out work-related activity increases from 8 to 17 per cent.[5]

Meanwhile, DWP is using every tool in its possession to prevent – or at least delay – the release of information from its peer reviews. In July 2015, the Information Commissioner's Office rules in DWP's favour, concluding that it had interpreted the legislation correctly. I appeal to the information rights tribunal, and rely on pro bono legal support provided by barrister Elizabeth Kelsey, of Monckton Chambers.

Campaigners secure a trickle of further information. DPAC's Annie Howard discovers that in ten of the 49 reviews the claimant who died had had their benefits sanctioned at some point, while journalist Natalie Leal is told that at least 22 of the claimants had been claiming ESA when they died. DWP tells me it 'does not hold information' on how it handles correspondence from coroners who express concern about the death of a benefit claimant. In

March 2016, it will send out a memo to 'all DWP business areas' to ensure that it now keeps a central record of correspondence from courts, coroners and (in Scotland) procurators fiscal and that these responses 'are correctly managed'. It refers to 'recent media interest' which 'has highlighted that the Department does not have sufficiently robust oversight of such correspondence'.

In April 2016, my peer review appeal reaches the information rights tribunal. It rules in my favour, thanks to Elizabeth Kelsey's astute legal advocacy. Tribunal judge Andrew Bartlett, who leads a three-person panel, says both DWP and the information commissioner had made an error in law in how they had interpreted Section 123 of the Social Security Administration Act 1992, which states that a civil servant is guilty of a criminal offence by disclosing 'without lawful authority any information which he acquired in the course of his employment and which relates to a particular person'. Bartlett agrees that they had interpreted the phrase 'relates to a particular person' too widely. He says there is material within the peer reviews that can be released, but only information not directly about those who died.

On 12 May, DWP finally releases redacted versions of the 49 peer reviews.[6] The only useful disclosures are the recommendations made by the reviews, but they still reveal vital information.

This is the first time any parts of the reviews have been published, and the redacted documents show where DWP's own investigations have concluded that improvements should be made locally or nationally. They show the department has been putting the lives of 'vulnerable' claimants at risk. In at least 13 reviews, the author explicitly raises concerns about the way such claimants were treated. The documents make it clear DWP was repeatedly warned that its WCA policies were risking lives.

One peer review – into the death of an incapacity benefit claimant who was being reassessed for ESA – stresses the costs of making the process safer. 'There is clearly a resource implication in treating more claimants with REDACTED as potentially vulnerable,' it says. 'However, that should be balanced against the resource implications of repeated appeals.'

Another says: 'The IB reassessment guidance … is not specific enough about the actions staff should take, once a claimant has been identified as vulnerable.'

At least four reviews include references to DWP staff failing to follow the six-point plan. The reviews all pre-date the suicide of Faiza Ahmed. One calls for 'further action to embed the Six Point Plan as it is a recurring theme'. Another uses almost exactly the same words.

The most shocking element of what emerges will only become clear in future years: that many of the flaws the newly released reviews reveal have not been fixed, and will continue to contribute to the deaths of countless disabled people.

Over the years researching these terrible deaths, the only time I have any chance of putting questions directly to DWP ministers is at the annual Conservative Party conference. And in October 2016, in Birmingham, I spot Iain Duncan Smith being interviewed by a regional broadcast journalist. After they finish, I approach Duncan Smith. (Some of his responses have not been included.)

JP: Hello, John Pring, from Disability News Service.
IDS: Oh yes.
JP: Can I have a quick word about Stephen Carré, the coroner's letter from 2010?
IDS: I can't remember that now.
JP: It would have been in your in-tray when you started. It was talking about further medical evidence, the WCA and that all people with mental health conditions needed to have further medical evidence as part of the WCA.
IDS: Back in 2010–11, Chris Grayling was in charge of it, he changed the nature of what we looked at. What we inherited from Labour at the time was quite a harsh system and we had if you remember about four or five reviews and each one of them recommended changes to soften it.
JP: But not on further medical evidence.
IDS: Particularly on mental health they did, yes.

JP: But not on further medical evidence. You'll remember there was a court case ...

...

JP: We're still waiting for that pilot project on the further medical evidence, the one that went through the high court and the Mental Health Resistance Network.

IDS: Yes, I don't know where the situation is now because I left back in March ... But the whole idea was to make it easier for people with mental health conditions to be able to establish the nature of their condition and the restrictions it placed upon them.

JP: But we are still waiting and people are still dying as a result ... and that's what the coroner suggested in that letter ...

IDS: Hold on. I'm not going to get in a debate with you because I don't know, I am not there anymore ... I'm now not there, so you need to talk to the department about where they are with that.

JP: You were secretary of state at the time.

IDS: I was ...

JP: And that letter was there in your inbox.

IDS: Yes, but the changes, the reviews, we had five reviews looking at this.

JP: Yes, but there was a prevention of further deaths report. It came from a coroner ...

IDS: We had five reviews and we have tried to make it easier for people with mental health. That's all I can say. I haven't got the details of it, so I can't ...

JP: Are you saying you don't remember the letter at all?

IDS: I remember the case and I remember the work we did and we had five reviews so I'm not going to be accused by you of anything, I'm simply saying ...

JP: It's the first time I've had the chance to ask you questions about it.

IDS: Yes, OK, well the reality is we have had five reviews ...

JP: You remember the letter?

IDS: I remember the early cases.

JP: You remember the letter from the coroner in 2010?

IDS: I can't remember every single letter from a coroner, I'm not ...

JP: It was a letter from a coroner about prevention of future deaths.

IDS: There were lots of issues around in the DWP at the time. I'm not going to say specifically in every case I can remember the details ...

JP: People have died since, such as Michael O'Sullivan, for instance.

IDS: Go and ask the department about where they are now with all of that. Honestly, because I am not there at the moment.

JP: You were there for five years.

IDS: Yes, I'm not there now, I'm not there now.

JP: Six years.

IDS: What I am saying to you is we did a lot to make it easier for them and that was worked on at the time. I'm simply saying to you it is better and easier than it was in 2010. And if you could acknowledge that that would be helpful.

JP: And about the Police Scotland situation?

IDS: I'm not there, I am not going to get involved in the detailed questioning from you because...

The interview was over.

The following month, Duncan Smith's bluster and misdirection are exposed when the UN committee on the rights of persons with disabilities – after taking evidence from Gill Thompson, Jill Gant, Anne-Marie O'Sullivan, and many disabled activists and allies – concludes the UK government is guilty of 'grave' and 'systematic' violations of disabled people's human rights.[7]

In the committee's first such inquiry, it finds that the government – mainly DWP – has discriminated against disabled people across three key parts of the UN Convention on the Rights of Persons with Disabilities. Disabled activists from DPAC – led by co-founder Debbie Jolly, who dies just days after the report is published – say it is a vindication of their four-year journey since asking the committee to investigate the government's actions in the name of austerity.

The report concludes that the reforms – including the introduction of the benefits cap and changes in eligibility criteria for personal independence payment – have 'disproportionately affected' disabled people, and that its evidence 'points to significant hardship, including financial, material and psychological' experienced by disabled people undergoing benefit assessments.

The government rejects all eleven recommendations and dismisses the report as 'patronising and offensive'.[8]

The following month DWP admits to me in a freedom of information response that there had been seven peer reviews that mentioned the work capability assessment in the period from February 2012 until Professor Malcolm Harrington submitted his final independent review of the assessment later that year. But when I ask how many were shared with Harrington, DWP replies: 'The Department does not hold any information to confirm or deny whether these Peer Reviews were shared with Professor Harrington.' There had been no mention of peer reviews into deaths linked to the WCA in any of his three independent reviews.

When I ask Professor Harrington whether he was shown these seven peer reviews – he has already told me he was not shown the Stephen Carré coroner's report – he emails me the following response:

> Dear John
>
> I can only repeat what I said to you earlier.
>
> I have NO recollection of seeing any of the reviews you mention.
>
> Maybe my brain is failing, but such damning indictments of the system – if seen – should have triggered a response from me.
>
> It didn't …
>
> So … maybe my memory serves me well after all!
>
> Kind regards,
>
> Malcolm

The evidence is slowly building, not only of the links between DWP reforms and the deaths of claimants, but of the department's repeated attempts to cover up those connections. Two months later, DWP tells the information commissioner it has destroyed records that would have shown how ten recommendations from the peer reviews were dealt with.[9] It says there is 'no requirement' for it to keep track of how it responds to recommendations, and has no legal duty to keep this information.

The information commissioner tells DWP she finds it 'unusual that a Central Government Department would dedicate resources to a process of case reviews and recommendations but not require the relevant departments to report back or record the actions taken in response to those recommendations'.

DWP claims it evaluated the system in April 2015 and made changes to 'improve accountability and responsibility and ensure that recommendations were identified, logged centrally and followed up so that outcomes were tracked, audited and understood'. Peer reviews were renamed 'internal process reviews' and all of them are now 'tracked centrally' with 'outcomes recorded'. A report by another public body, three years later, will show these claims to be completely untrue.

20

The Death of Jodey Whiting

All her family have stories about Jodey as a child.

About a seven-year-old Jodey and her cousin Stu finding a goat and bringing it back to her nana's house and Jodey saying she wanted to adopt it.

The day the family hired a boat on holiday in Corfu and Jodey took the wheel and immediately opened the throttle as far as it would go. They are all knocked to the floor, the boat bouncing over the waves. 'We all thought we were going to drown,' her dad, Eric, would say later.

The time Jodey and her best friend Debbie were given money to have their hair done; they cut each other's hair themselves and kept the money for cigarettes.

Jodey could make friends with anyone, says her mum, Joy Dove. She loves animals, and is obsessed with her dolls. She fusses over her brother Jamie when he is born, and when older she loves babysitting for local families, and can often be seen with a trail of children tagging along in her wake. But she also struggles to concentrate and pay attention in class, and there are tantrums, mood swings, anxiety, meltdowns. She is accident-prone. She ends up in A&E with a dog bite, and gets a pencil stuck into her cheek while playing behind the sofa.

Donna, older by two years, is the swot, while Jodey plays truant. 'We were polar opposites,' says Donna. 'My earliest memory of being at nana's was that Jodey got me to open my mouth and she squirted bleach in my mouth, and I had to be rushed to hospital. She had these beautiful blue eyes, but she was like a little tornado.'

Her brother Jamie, younger by six years, remembers winding Jodey up and standing at the top of the stairs. 'She was behind me and pushed me down the stairs. Sometimes it would be great, but sometimes we would fight like cat and dog. But if anyone picked on me, she would be right there,' he says. He remembers moving up to secondary school, and being picked on by an older girl. Jodey, who by now had left school and was heavily pregnant, marched down to the school and went looking for the girl. Jamie could hear doors slamming in the corridors as his sister searched for the bully.

Jodey is adored by her family, and she is caring and kind – she visits Joy in hospital every day when she is ill – but she is also impulsive and challenging to parent. She often goes missing, and when she is 15 and has become almost unmanageable, she asks to go into care. After just ten days, she decides to come home.

Jodey leaves school at 16 after becoming pregnant, and moves into a council house in Thornaby. There are no curtains, so she pastes newspapers on the windows. But she runs out and sticks up pages ripped out of porn magazines. 'Everyone was talking about that house,' says Jamie. 'That's the kind of person she was. She just couldn't give a crap.'

Jodey's physical health problems begin with curvature of the spine, which is first noticeable as a teenager. In her early 20s, the back pain begins to worsen, with numerous hospital treatments and operations over the next 20 years. She is eventually diagnosed with Klippel-Feil Syndrome, a fusion of bones in the neck. She takes ever more painkillers.

She marries Martin – known as Belly – when she is 18. Her family remember Jodey charging into a takeaway for chips on the way to the wedding. They have nine children by her late 20s, including two sets of twins. In one year, she has a baby in January and then twins in October; another year she has twins in November and another baby eleven months later. Belly works as a care assistant in a nursing home; Jodey works there briefly before her childcare duties take over. She loves her children, and they become – and remain – the centre of her life.

But Jodey's mental health begins to deteriorate. She first has contact with the crisis team in her mid-20s, and that will continue – off and on – for the rest of her life, but the lack of regular input from a professional she can learn to trust means there is rarely any improvement. 'Sometimes she would sleep for a few days because of the medication and the pain and then she would be awake for a few days,' says Donna, 'and then she would crash again.'

Jodey is told she has bipolar but is later diagnosed with borderline personality disorder and then with emotionally unstable personality disorder. There are frequent suicide attempts, including at least nine between 2009 and 2015.

In her mid-30s, Belly leaves her. It has a significant impact on Jodey's mental health. She is not well enough to look after her children permanently, so they live with their dad. For a while, she lives in hostels, but still sees her children.

Her love for her family is unquestionable. The birthday and other greetings-cards she sends are filled with affection. 'We love you loads, you're the best mam in the world and I will never forget that,' she writes in a card Joy still treasures.

As her health deteriorates, it becomes increasingly difficult for Jodey to leave her home. The medication has caused cirrhosis and other side-effects, including problems with her teeth. Joy becomes her carer – arranging her daughter's bills, shopping, doctor's appointments, and official letters.

Jodey is now living in a flat in Hume House, a high-rise on the edge of Stockton. She is rarely well enough to leave the third-floor flat. There are black blinds on the windows, black chandeliers, and pictures of Marilyn Monroe and Audrey Hepburn.

She had been claiming incapacity benefit and income support between 2006 and 2012, but is reassessed for ESA in 2012. She has a face-to-face assessment, with an Atos healthcare professional recording her severe mental distress and concluding her health would be at risk if found fit for work. The report is passed to DWP, which awards Jodey ESA for two years, placing her in the support group. An electronic flag is placed on the system, which means a form should automatically be sent to her GP to request medical evidence when she is reassessed.

She is sent another ESA50 questionnaire two years later, on which she writes: 'Most days I want to kill myself, if my doctor doesn't get the pain under control asap I plan 2 kill myself.'

The mental health flag means Atos requests further evidence from her GP, who confirms on 8 September 2014 that Jodey has a long-standing diagnosis of emotionally unstable personality disorder, with constant stress, low mood, and anxiety. She is again found not fit for work, this time without the need for a face-to-face assessment.

Her family encourage Jodey to wean herself off the pills. 'She had been on that much medication that she said it didn't touch her,' says Donna. 'She was sleeping in her front room. She couldn't leave the flat. She was like a prisoner.'

Jodey wants to buy a mobility scooter, but she can't afford one because DWP has cut her personal independence payment.

It is 2016. Jodey has been struggling with pneumonia and a gastric condition. She is admitted to hospital with gastritis and duodenitis, inflammation of her intestines. Later, still experiencing a persistent cough, she needs a chest x-ray. Over the next few months, there are concerns about possible abuse of medication, and continuing back pain. She mentions to hospital staff a persistent pain behind her ears and her eye. A scan finds a benign cyst on her brain. She returns home to convalesce.

DWP sends her another ESA50 questionnaire. She requests a home visit, writing: 'I have suicidal thoughts a lot of the time and could not cope with work or looking for work.' Again, a mental health flag is raised on the system.

But DWP fails to refer Jodey's request for a home assessment to Maximus. Maximus also fails to consider the request once it receives her ESA50 form. But it does send a form to Jodey's GP to request further medical evidence. The GP confirms Jodey was referred to the mental health crisis team in June for intensive treatment due to suicidal thoughts, and was discharged ten days later as 'nil suicide intent/thoughts', but provides little useful information about her lengthy history of mental distress.

On 15 December, Maximus concludes that Jodey needs to attend a face-to-face assessment, and writes to ask her to visit the Thornaby assessment centre on 16 January. Jodey is now on eight different medications, 23 tablets a day, including two lots of morphine, a tranquiliser, anti-anxiety medication, and two anti-depressants.

The Maximus letter has been stuck in a drawer with many other brown envelopes, so Jodey misses the assessment. DWP asks her in writing to explain why she failed to attend. DWP guidance states it should have phoned her to check why she missed the assessment, but an investigation later finds no evidence this was done. DWP should also have considered a safeguarding visit. Again, the investigation finds no evidence of this.

When Jodey returns the form on 24 January, she tells DWP: 'I did not receive the appointment letter and I have been housebound with pneumonia been in hospital and I found out I have cyst of the brain.' She says she did not receive a phone call. She says her GP wants DWP to request information on her medical background, but no contact is made.

Joy helps her daughter with the form, and they enclose evidence of her medication. They are sure everything will be OK, once DWP knows about the hospital treatment, the cyst on the brain, and the pneumonia. But DWP writes back two weeks later to say Jodey is now considered fit for work because she has not shown good cause for failing to attend the WCA. The decision-maker says she has not provided any medical proof of the pneumonia. The letter makes no reference to her mental health.

Jodey phones DWP on 10 February and is told to secure medical evidence and seek a 'mandatory reconsideration'. She does this on 13 February and states again that she is unable to work, adding: 'Please reconsider and send or ring new appointment for me.'

DWP's letter causes her immense distress. 'It was unbelievable,' says her mum. 'Jodey was crying. She said, "What am I going to do, mam? I can't walk out the door, I can't breathe, let alone sign on."'

'The flat was a haven for her and she thought she was going to lose it,' says Donna. Jodey knows she cannot work, or cope without the ESA.

They seek help from the local Citizens Advice Bureau, which on 15 February helps them draft a letter to DWP, requesting a home visit and a review of the decision. The letter points out Jodey's depression and anxiety and that she is not always able to deal with her post, while she takes large quantities of painkillers that affect her concentration. She would have attended the assessment if she had known about it, the letter says, and asks for another WCA. Only now does she finally open the letter that told her to attend the WCA. Citizens Advice sends her letter to DWP. The department will claim it was never received. An investigation will later conclude that DWP missed five opportunities 'to prompt particular consideration' of her mental health and 'give careful consideration to her case because of it'.

Jodey writes to her GP, to tell him how worried she is about her benefits being stopped and to ask for a letter to pass to DWP, but he is on holiday, and no one else at the surgery can help.

While they are waiting for DWP to consider the mandatory reconsideration, further letters arrive, this time telling her that, because her ESA is stopping, so too are her housing benefit and council tax support.

Jodey begins to talk about dying, telling Joy: 'If anything happens, don't be screaming.' And she tells her brother: 'If anything happens to us, don't worry.' The family think she is worrying about her physical health.

On 19 February, Jodey says she is feeling suicidal and calls the mental health crisis team. They offer her a place at a mental health unit. She has been there before and rejects the offer.

The next day, Joy phones DWP, asking if her daughter can apply for a crisis loan. They tell her Jodey will have to go to the jobcentre. Joy tells Jodey about the possibility of a loan. Jodey isn't well enough to visit the jobcentre, so Joy goes instead. 'They have a worker stood at the front door with a security guard,' Joy would say later. 'You have to get past this worker, who either says, "OK, sit and wait" or you have to leave. But she said, "No, the case is dormant. She'll have to sign on." She didn't even allow me to go and sit down and discuss it with the worker on the computer.'

When Joy tells her daughter, Jodey's face falls. 'What am I gonna do? I can't walk out the door, I can't breathe.' She begins to cry.

'Jodey, don't worry,' says Joy. 'If we don't get your money back, if we don't get it sorted, I'll go up the Gazette.' The *Gazette* is their local paper.

Jodey's daughter Emma has asked her mum to stay with her until she hears the result of her mandatory reconsideration. Emma realises her mum needs extra support, and texts her later, asking her: 'Are you still coming over, mam?' Jodey's last words to her daughter are: 'I'm going to sleep … I love you and the girls.' Emma tries ringing her all evening but there is no answer. She thinks her mum has gone to bed.

Joy speaks to Jodey, who tells her she will be staying with Emma the next day. Her last words are: 'I love you, mam. I'm going to sleep.'

The next day, Jodey has not called or texted. Joy assumes she is at Emma's. When she phones Jodey at tea-time, there is no answer. Joy phones Emma, who tells her: 'She's not here, nana.'

Joy panics. She phones the concierge and asks him to ring the buzzer to Jodey's flat. There is no answer. Joy, several miles away at her flat in Norton, phones the police. 'We knew she wouldn't be out of the flat. She hadn't got the strength to walk out,' she would tell me later. Officers visit Jodey's flat. Joy phones after an hour, and is told the officers knocked on Jodey's door, but no one answered. They left when they received a 999 call.

Meanwhile, Emma takes a taxi, picks up her younger sister Amy, and heads to Hume House. The concierge won't let them in. 'I was begging them, crying, saying, "please, I know something's wrong with her, I know,"' Emma will later tell a *Dispatches* documentary for Channel 4.

Eventually, they manage to enter the building when a resident comes out. They bang on their mum's door and look through the letterbox. 'I knew something was wrong, you could just feel it,' said Emma. Emma calls Joy and asks her to bring a spare key. When she arrives, the key won't work. The concierge helps her open the door. He walks into the flat ahead of Joy and her two granddaughters.

When the concierge turns on the light, Joy sees Jodey sitting upright on the sofa, with her hands resting on her legs. Joy falls against the wall and starts to scream, saying: 'Jodey, no, please, wake up, Jodey, wake up.' Amy also begins screaming, and stumbles into the bathroom to be sick. Emma is the last to see her mum on the sofa.

One of Jodey's eyes is shut. A single tear has run down from the other eye. 'I've got to her, I've touched her, she's stone cold,' Emma would tell *Dispatches*. She begs her mum to wake up. Amy has collapsed on the floor and is trying to phone her dad.

On the sofa is a blue notebook, decorated with a ribbon, that Jodey bought in a post-Christmas sale. Inside it, she has written messages for each of her children, and for Joy.

In her note to her mother, Jodey has written: 'MAM, I love u so much, you r my ledgend, plz keep my baby's safe plz mam, always watch ova them, I'm at peace with nana's, I will always watch ova u all, believe me xx.'

Joy finds other observations in the notebook that show her daughter's desperation, often just a few scribbled words. There is a mixture of concern for her children, frustration with her health conditions, and always – running like a dark thread through the notebook – her money problems.

'Could n pay bills … breathless – bk pain … trying to pay bills … head hurts,' she writes.

And: 'I cnt cope no more … I've had enough.'

Then: 'debt debt debt'.

Joy decides to fight for justice for her daughter. She calls the *Gazette*, just as she promised Jodey she would, and speaks to chief reporter Ian Johnson. He has recently covered the story of a young man who took his own life 'under immense pressure' from jobcentre staff who told him his benefits would be stopped unless he did more to find work. He promises to cover the inquest.

The inquest happens quickly, on 24 May, just three months after Jodey's death. The verdict is suicide, but Joy is frustrated at the failure to take evidence from DWP. She had tried to raise her concerns with the coroner's office in Middlesbrough, arguing in two letters that she believed DWP pushed her daughter to take her own life. Her letters are read out, but there is no probing of DWP's role in Jodey's death, and there are no DWP witnesses.

Joy gives brief oral evidence, and confirms that having her ESA stopped was a factor in Jodey's death. Emma tells the inquest: 'They knew my mam off a screen … because of their wrong choice, we've lost our best friend.' Joy says she is fighting for her daughter and wants 'justice for Jodey'.

The hearing lasts just 37 minutes. The coroner mentions the ESA claim and the family's concerns, but says it is not for the inquest to investigate or comment upon DWP's failings, or question its decisions. She rules that Jodey took her own life, but there is no criticism of the department.

Ian Johnson has attended the inquest. Joy tells him the department 'has blood on their hands'. The next day, the story is on the *Gazette*'s front page.

* * *

In the same week, and nearly five years after the high court granted permission for a judicial review of DWP's WCA failures, we finally learn the pitiful measures the department has taken, after years of its delays, obstruction, and misdirection.

They only emerge in response to freedom of information requests from Disability News Service and Public Law Project (PLP), which represents the two anonymous claimants who took the case.

Existing DWP guidance says further medical evidence (FME) 'should always be requested' if there is 'evidence of risk of suicide or self-harm expressed in the questionnaire, previous reports or any documentation relating to the case'. But further medical evidence can also now be requested if it is felt that 'further information would be helpful'. But if the healthcare professional decides to seek this FME, 'the reason must be clearly justified and documented'.

This is a tiny improvement, but nowhere near the demand made by the Mental Health Resistance Network – which backed the legal case – PLP and Professor Malcolm Harrington, that Maximus should 'actively consider the need to seek further documentary evidence in every claimant's case', and that any decision not to seek further evidence 'must be justified', with 'particular care' to be taken to ensure this evidence is obtained when the claimant has a mental health condition or learning difficulty. PLP says DWP's response 'must call into question whether there is any political will to stop the discriminatory effect of the WCA' on people in mental distress.

The same question has to be asked of parliament. Although a handful of Labour and SNP backbenchers have raised concerns, the work and pensions committee – with its Labour chairs but Conservative majorities – has done little to expose the links between DWP and countless deaths.

In December 2017, not yet aware of Jodey's death, I publish some startling figures.[1] They show that in 2007 – a year before the introduction of the work capability assessment – 21 per cent of incapacity benefit (IB) claimants said they had attempted suicide at some point in their lives. By 2014, six years after WCA was introduced, and following four years of coalition cuts and reforms, more than 43 per cent of claimants were saying they had attempted suicide at some point. Over the same period, attempted suicide figures for adults who were not claiming IB (in 2007) or ESA (in 2014) had remained statistically stable (6.0 per cent in 2007 against 6.7 per cent in 2014).

The analysis has been carried out by Sally McManus, who leads research on the Adult Psychiatric Morbidity Survey for the social research institute NatCen, on behalf of NHS Digital. These figures do not prove the WCA and austerity reforms caused a rapid increase in attempted suicides, particularly because the IB and ESA populations will have been different, but one leading psychologist and disabled activist, Dr Jay Watts, tells me the figures show 'the greatest increase in suicide rates for any population that I can recall in the literature'.

Despite being aware of the startling figures from the 2014 survey, which had been published in September 2016, the government refuses to explain why it failed to prioritise ESA claimants as a high-risk group for suicide in its latest suicide prevention strategy.

The week after I publish the figures, members of the work and pensions committee – chaired by Labour's former DWP minister Frank Field – refuse to ask the new minister for disabled people, Sarah Newton, about the figures when she is questioned as part of an inquiry into benefit assessments. 'How is it possible that the minister for disabled people was not asked about the doubling of attempted suicide rates so clearly linked to the policies of her department?' Jay Watts asks afterwards. Denise McKenna, co-founder of the Mental Health Resistance Network, describes this failure as a 'dereliction of duty by the whole committee'.

Meanwhile, Joy Dove has been working with Citizens Advice to appeal the decision on Jodey's benefits. Within two weeks of her death, it is overturned. But Joy wants to take her concerns further and lodges a complaint with the independent case examiner (ICE), which examines complaints against DWP.

I speak to Joy for the first time in April 2018. An activist has confronted work and pensions secretary Esther McVey about Jodey's death as she was giving evidence to the Scottish parliament's social security committee. The activist, sitting behind McVey, called to her: 'What about Jodey Whiting, mother of nine, who committed suicide after her ESA was stopped? It was stopped because she missed an appointment.'

Joy, who has arranged a Justice for Jodey petition that demands a change in the law and an inquiry, tells me she was delighted to hear how the activist confronted McVey, which she sees as another step in her campaign for justice for her daughter. 'I have kept strong for my daughter,' she says, 'but I am heartbroken, I always will be.' She says she spends many tearful hours by Jodey's grave, quietly filling her daughter in on family news.

She writes to prime minister Theresa May to ask for a meeting, but her request is dismissed because of 'the tremendous pressures of her diary'. The letter makes no mention of Jodey and expresses no condolences.

In May 2018, about a year after Jodey's death, DWP tells me in a freedom of information response that it has no record of whether it showed vital documents linking the work capability assessment with the deaths of claimants to Dr Paul Litchfield, who had published the final two reviews of the WCA in December 2013 and November 2014.

The missing documents included at least seven peer reviews that mentioned the WCA and the two prevention of future deaths (PFD) reports written by coroners following the suicides of Stephen Carré and Michael O'Sullivan. The existence of these documents had only been revealed publicly in the years after Litchfield's final report was published. Neither of his reports mentioned peer reviews or PFD reports. Professor Malcom Harrington, who carried out the first three reviews of the WCA, has already told me he is convinced that DWP did not show him either the relevant peer reviews or the Stephen Carré PFD report.

The evidence is mounting that DWP hid evidence from both of its independent reviewers that linked the WCA with the deaths of benefit claimants.

* * *

Joy receives the ICE report in February 2019. It reveals how DWP failed five times to follow its own safeguarding rules in the weeks leading to Jodey's suicide. Joy calls for DWP and those staff responsible to face a criminal investigation, and says her daughter died a 'martyr' and that campaigners are right to say the government has created a 'hostile environment for disabled people'.

The independent case examiner, Joanna Wallace, says: 'In total there have been five opportunities for DWP processes to prompt particular consideration of Jodey's mental health status and give careful consideration to her case because of it – none of those were taken.' DWP agrees to pay £10,000 to the family as a 'consolatory' payment for its 'repeated failures to follow their safeguarding procedures', and other failings that took place after Jodey's death.

After the ICE ruling, I help Joy find a solicitor. Eventually, thanks to assistance from organisations such as Public Law Project and Inquest, solicitors Leigh Day take on the legal fight for a second inquest, one that would examine DWP's failings in depth.

The following month, Joy's is one of six families who support a parliamentary petition[2] I've drawn up, backed by a series of grassroots groups of disabled people, including DPAC, Black Triangle, the Mental Health Resistance Network, WOW campaign, and the disabled women's organisation WinVisible. The petition calls for an independent inquiry, for evidence of misconduct to be passed to the police, brands DWP 'institutionally disablist and not fit for purpose', and calls on the department to urgently 'make the safety of all claimants a priority'. The petition is also backed by Peter Carré, Jill Gant, David Barr, Gill Thompson, and Eleanor Donnachie, who lost her brother Paul to suicide after his ESA was removed when he failed to turn up for an assessment.

Three months later, Joy and Eric are visited by Emma Haddad, DWP's director general for service excellence, and Colin Stewart, its work and health director for the north of England. Joy asks a series of questions I have drafted for her, but Haddad refuses to answer most of them for 'legal reasons'. 'It hasn't really changed things because she's dead and she's not coming back,' Joy says afterwards. 'I told them that five minutes away from here, my daughter is in that cemetery.'

On 13 March, Theresa May is asked about the ICE ruling by Joy's MP, Dr Paul Williams, in prime minister's questions.[3] She expresses sympathy, admits there were mistakes, and says DWP is looking at the case 'to ensure that we never see such failings happening again and leading to such a tragic consequence'.

But DWP has no interest in making the changes necessary to end the slow, creeping violence. By now, harm is built into the institution, into its buildings, its software, its management, and its policies.

* * *

Over the years, Joy agrees to multiple media interviews, including an appearance on Victoria Derbyshire's BBC show. She speaks at the *Daily Mirror*'s Labour conference fringe event in Brighton in September 2019, and receives a standing ovation.

She also takes part in an action by disabled artist-activist Dolly Sen outside DWP's Caxton House offices in Westminster. She and others hold up heart-shaped boards, on which are written the names of Jodey, Stephen Carré, Mark Wood, and Susan Roberts, whose deaths were all closely linked to DWP. Other hearts show the phrases 'broken hearts for the DWP' and 'hearts stopped by DWP policies'. 'We will fight for every person who is let down by the building behind us,' says Dolly. As DWP staff enter and leave the building, she asks each of them if they will sign off the next death to be caused by DWP. They all ignore her. 'When I saw the heart I wanted to cry,' Joy tells me, 'but I had to be strong for Jodey.' It was her first visit to London since 1983. It won't be her last.

Joy writes a book, *A Mother's Job*,[4] with authors Ann and Joe Cusack, which follows both her own journey from 'passive and easy-going' great-grandmother to fierce campaigner, and Jodey's story. She still lights a candle for her daughter each night in a shrine of mementos in her flat and – when she is at her lowest – sprays Jodey's favourite deodorant so she can feel close to her.

* * *

In November 2020, Joy hears that the solicitor general, Michael Ellis, has granted her permission to ask the high court to order a second inquest. The case reaches the high court in June 2021. But despite nearly a decade of high-profile tragedies, legal cases, research, television exposés, and parliamentary debates, government barrister David Griffiths insists the flaws that led to Jodey's death were not part of a 'systemic' problem but due to individual errors. If there was such a 'systemic problem', he says, it would be 'known and public to a great extent'. He assures the judges that DWP would have told the court if there was any indication of a systemic problem.

When the court delivers its ruling, in September 2021, it refuses to quash the result of the first inquest. Mrs Justice Farbey argues that DWP's failings had been 'shocking' but its errors 'amounted to individual failings attributable to mistakes or bad judgment' and were not 'systemic or structural in nature'. In October 2022, the Court of Appeal grants Joy permission to appeal.

The following March, the court delivers its ruling:[5] it is 'in the interests of justice' for there to be another inquest. Lady Justice Whipple, one of three appeal judges, says the extent to which DWP's actions contributed to Jodey's mental health deteriorating 'is a matter of real significance to Mrs Dove and her family' and it is 'reasonable for them to press for that matter to be investigated as part of the inquest into Jodey's death', while there is a 'wider public interest' in the coroner considering what caused Jodey's mental health to deteriorate.

Joy says it is a victory not just for her family but for all those mourning relatives whose deaths have been linked to the department's actions and for 'others still on the receiving end of awful treatment by the DWP'.

In November 2023, a pre-inquest review takes place at Teesside Magistrates' Court in Middlesbrough. Senior coroner Clare Bailey promises there will now be a 'full and fearless' inquest.[6] Joy's daughter Donna tells me: 'I have watched my mam crying her eyes out in the first video interview she did, and then gone from that to this warrior woman. What she's done, it amazes me.'

People keep coming up to Joy and telling her how strong she is. But she's not as strong as they think. She is referred for counselling after a return of the depression and anxiety that first affected her as an 18-year-old mum. She resorts to obsessive-compulsive 'little rituals' – washing her hands ten times, repeatedly brushing her hair. She doesn't sleep well, waking every hour. She puts an extra pillow on her bed, putting her arm around it as though Jodey is still there with her.

21

The Death of James Oliver

She sits, almost cross-legged, right up against the microphone so she can hold it between her toes. Theresia Degener, professor of law and disability studies and chair of the UN committee on the rights of persons with disabilities, is delivering one of the strongest public condemnations of the government and its austerity years.

She stares at the UK delegation as she tells them the cuts to social security and other support have caused 'a human catastrophe' which is 'totally neglecting the vulnerable situation' disabled people are in.[1] Representatives of disabled people's organisations have travelled to Geneva to provide detailed evidence for the examination of the government's progress in implementing the UN Convention on the Rights of Persons with Disabilities.

Another committee member, Stig Langvad, says it has 'become evident that the committee has a very different perception of how human rights should be understood and implemented' than the UK government. 'I could provide a long list of examples where the state party doesn't live up to the convention,' he says. 'Unfortunately, the time is too limited.'

The human catastrophe continues to play out. Since its launch in 2013, many of the same concerns raised about the WCA are now being levelled at the new assessment for personal independence payment (PIP). PIP is replacing disability living allowance for working-age claimants as a contribution to the many extra costs disabled people face, such as their need for mobility equipment, extra heating and washing costs, special diets, and the need for support around the house.

But concerns have been growing about the PIP assessments. Over eight months, I collect more than 200 cases in which disabled people describe how assessors have lied in their written assessment reports. Despite this evidence, DWP and its contractors refuse to investigate the claims of widespread dishonesty.[2] Those contractors are Atos and Capita. Capita was formed in 1987 from a management buyout of the consultancy arm of the Chartered Institute of Public Finance, and became the 'company of choice' to run many of New Labour's 'pet projects' in the 2000s.[3] DWP's refusal to address these concerns will, just as with the WCA, have tragic consequences.

* * *

James Oliver has been reliant on alcohol since he was eleven. It is how he copes with what his brother describes as a 'terrible childhood', with a step-dad who was 'a cruel, bullying, wife-beating thug'. Dave coped by withdrawing from society. James used drink and drugs. He was a charmer, who was always in trouble as a child. After school, which he leaves with a handful of CSEs, James works hard in a succession of jobs, often as a labourer, and for a few years in Amsterdam. His alcoholism pushes away family and friends, and wrecks a succession of relationships.

His final job is with a bakery, a job he loves. But when the business closes, and his body begins to break down after years of alcohol abuse, he must rely on the state.

On 17 April 2018, an Atos nurse visits James in his ground-floor flat in St-Leonards-on-Sea. James had applied for the second time for PIP, having been rejected two years earlier after being assessed by a paramedic. For the last two years he has needed regular blood transfusions.

James's organs have been destroyed by a lifetime of heavy drinking. His inability to look after himself, his almost-constant pain and discomfort, and his desperate need for financial support, should be obvious to the nurse as she takes out her laptop and begins asking questions about the challenges he faces when cooking, cleaning, maintaining his personal hygiene, using the toilet, and with his mobility.

In the centre of the room is a large wooden table, piled with packets of medication, many of them unopened. Citalopram, Zopiclone, Ramipril, Omeprazole, and the vitamin thiamine. The table surface is thick with dust, and there is an ashtray full of cigarette butts. So much dog hair is embedded in the carpet that when his brother later tries to vacuum the flat, he blows five fuses before conceding defeat. In the kitchen, the oven is encrusted with rust and months-old burnt food. There is blood in the sink and the bath. In the bedroom, the mattress is now yellow, and stained with blood and faeces. Dave will later describe the flat as 'like a dungeon'.

His daily routine involves a long, tortuous walk to Lidl with Hachi, a black, white and tan Alsatian cross he rescued from Bulgaria. It is about half a mile each way but can take more than two hours. He stocks up on cans of beer or cider and a few bags of crisps or sausage rolls. Without a car, or – thanks to DWP's decision in 2016 to deny him PIP – the money to pay for a taxi, he can only manage a few items. The staff at Lidl know him well and help him find food that is on offer.

Although a close inspection of the flat is not within the nurse's remit, the grim living conditions are obvious. The written evidence James provided should have been equally persuasive. 'I sometimes don't even eat as I forget to do so,' he writes on the PIP form. 'I have to remind myself to take my pills as I am getting very forgetful and have to remind myself what ones I have taken.'

He also writes of his constant sickness, and how that affects his personal hygiene: 'I bath once a week. Can't use perfumed products or I start coughing and being sick.' He uses baby-wipes to clean himself because of the constant diarrhoea, and often has to throw away his underwear because of his double incontinence. 'I can't eat hot food because I'm straight in the toilet. If I'm out I need to be always near a toilet or I foul myself.' He never ties his shoelaces because he becomes breathless when he leans down.

He lives a solitary life. 'I don't talk to anyone and I generally stay indoors,' he writes. 'I don't like people … I keep to myself and ignore my front door as much as I can.' The seriousness of his health conditions is clear. 'I keep ending up in hospital throwing up blood and bowel blood to (sic) I have just been discharged after having 3 blood transfusions.' Walking is also a trial. 'I get short of breath and so I can't walk far without stopping. I have got two walking sticks as I do have problems with my knees and can't go far without resting or needing to go to the toilet.' His brother would say later that James would tire himself out walking to the kitchen, and would come back drenched in sweat.

None of this is enough for the nurse. Her report briskly dismisses the pain, the discomfort, the breathlessness, the double incontinence. There is nothing about the state of the flat. She reports how James answered the door and claims he used a walking stick at a 'normal pace' and with 'normal gait'. 'He did not appear to put any weight on the walking stick. He stood from the chair without difficulty … He was seen alone and was talkative and laughed throughout the assessment … He appeared well kempt, clean and appropriately dressed. He was observed to be drinking cider during the assessment but did not appear in a drunken state.' He looks well, she writes.

'He reports he can walk for 5 minutes with a walking stick at a slow pace before needing to rest due to pain in his back and knee,' she writes. 'He reports he will walk to his local shop which takes 30–45 minutes and he will rest every 5 minutes. He reports he can potter around at home for 5 minutes at a time.' She also writes: 'He reports he can manage his own toilet needs, wipe himself and has no incontinence.' She describes how he has reported 'no pain' and 'did not appear breathless'. Although it is not her decision on whether James should be granted PIP, the outcome is inevitable.

The DWP decision-maker awards James zero points for every one of the independent living and mobility descriptors. The decision suggests James has been lying: 'At the consultation, there was no evidence of a significant physical restriction. There was no sign of breathlessness and you did not appear in pain… I have decided you can prepare and cook a simple meal for one person unaided… manage medication or therapy or monitor your health condition unaided, wash and bathe unaided, manage your toilet needs or incontinence unaided, dress and undress unaided.'

It is a similar conclusion with mobility. 'At the consultation there was no evidence of a significant physical restriction. There was no sign of breathlessness and you did not appear in pain. You were observed to walk at a normal pace and gait… I have decided you can stand and then move more than 200 metres.'

James asks for a mandatory reconsideration – essentially the first-stage appeal – and attaches a letter. He says he has found the PIP decision 'hard to come to terms with as I have lots of medical conditions and [am] taking countless prescriptions to help me'. He says he feels 'angry' and 'let down'. 'Some of the things I have to deal with on a daily basis are sciatica, constant trips to the toilet (at least 15 times a day) … unable to have proper hygine as once in the bath fear I'm unable to get back out. As with the toilet visits most times I don't make it and soil myself and when its blood this can be very upsetting.'

He adds: 'Your colleague that came to see me only sat there and took note on the laptop they had, they know nothing of my conditions and seemed unable to understand my everyday life. As in your letter you might want to get the facts of my case right before you decide that I am not "worthy".'

His appeal, and the letter, are rejected. Again, he is scored zero for all twelve descriptors. He secures some welfare rights advice, from Hastings Advice and Representation Centre (HARC). The next stage is to appeal to a tribunal. HARC encloses a letter from one of its advisers, detailing the points she believes James should have been awarded: 25 points for independent living, and 20 for mobility. This would have been enough to entitle him to the enhanced rate of PIP for both independent living and mobility.

* * *

James and Dave had drifted apart, but in the last few years they are reconciled, and Dave can provide some support, and help his brother with groceries every now and then. There are limits, though, because Dave himself has had a brain haemorrhage. 'He never used to be a person who cried,' said Dave later. 'But in those last 18 months I saw him cry a lot and it was always about the DWP and how cruel they were being.'

Several months after his claim is rejected, James begins to feel particularly unwell as he returns from his daily struggle to walk to Lidl. The walk back with his dog Hachi is a series of stops and starts. It is downhill, at least, but today it is even slower than usual. Eventually, he stumbles, staggers, and falls to the pavement. When the ambulance arrives, the blood has run 30 feet down the pavement.

James is rushed to hospital, but it is clear he doesn't have long left to live. Dave visits him in his hospital bed and is shocked by his condition. His skin is yellow with jaundice. He tells Dave: 'I can't believe I'm going to die and I'm still not sick enough for personal independence payment.'

'That was the day before he passed away,' said Dave. 'He'd been told the previous year that he was going to die and it was upsetting him, so he began to buck his ideas up a bit and he went into low alcohol drinks.' If he kept to the beers and avoided the spirits, he might have another twelve to 18 months, he was told. But when his PIP was rejected again by DWP it 'pushed him over the edge'. 'It dominated every conversation I had with him,' said Dave. 'It was always about the DWP and how they didn't care and they just wanted him to die. Once he'd gone into hospital they couldn't get enough blood into him.' It was too late. His body had given up.

A picture of the two of them taken as James lies in his hospital bed shows him smiling for the camera, although it is more of a grimace. Dave's white hair and the clean hospital bedlinen are a striking contrast to James's jaundiced skin.

James dies at about 6am on Tuesday 9 April. His family arrive half an hour too late. He leaves four sons and two daughters. James is 49, but as his brother will say later, he looks ten to 15 years older. As Dave left the ward for the last time, his brother had said: 'I love you.'

'I love you, too,' Dave replied.

'I knew that was the end because he never said I love you – ever,' Dave would say later. 'I'm glad we had that time together. I think we needed it. I tried to have a bit of a laugh with him because it was quite obvious that he wasn't going to be there for long. He'd spoken to the consultant that day and he said, "you haven't got long at all," and he'd cried that morning. But even that last day the DWP was still at the forefront of his mind, because they had basically taken over his mind since 2016 when he first tried to claim. There were tubes everywhere. The hospital staff couldn't move him without causing him pain. Everything hurt. And yet ... still no PIP.'

Dave launches a Facebook campaign, and a petition[4] calling on the government to scrap the outsourcing of assessments to private contractors. 'There would be some justice for his sons and daughters,' he says, 'if private companies were no longer involved in these assessments, and the DWP looked at the client from beginning to end with their own specialist. That would give me some peace of mind that his death wasn't in vain, nor the death of all the others.'

Dave is, in his own words, 'the least likely person ever to get involved in something like this. I never wanted my face on TV or in the papers and yet I let all this happen because I began to think that this needs to be seen. And that's when I began to learn how bad this whole situation is. It's bullying, but bullying beyond belief. Discrimination doesn't come close. It's just violent, what they're doing.'

He works through his brother's paperwork, highlighting the inaccuracies and the lies in the assessment reports. 'If this was a company with this many deaths on its hands,' Dave tells me, 'it would be forced to cease trading and have a criminal inquiry. All the promises of "it will never happen again" by the DWP are a total waste of time because it is a department which doesn't know how to behave in a humane way.'

In a rare case of DWP admitting its errors, a spokesperson tells me the department is 'very sorry for the distress caused and are looking into this to prevent it happening again'. But DWP insists it has made 'significant improvements' to its assessments.

Only weeks earlier, Disability News Service revealed that disabled people were now almost twice as likely to win their disability benefit appeal than ten years earlier, at the start of almost a decade of austerity-era Conservative control of DWP. The proportion of tribunal appeals that found in favour of disability living allowance claimants was just 38 per cent in 2010–11, the first year of the Conservative-Liberal Democrat coalition. But the rate of tribunal success[5] for PIP claimants has risen from 26 per cent in 2013–14, to 50 per cent in 2014–15, to 61 per cent the following year, and then to 73 per cent of PIP claimants by 2018–19, almost twice the rate of success of DLA claimants in 2010–11.

DWP argues that only about 4 or 5 per cent of PIP claims are eventually appealed successfully. But most successful claimants don't appeal, for obvious reasons, and many rejected claimants do not challenge the decision, with DWP's own research[6] showing that hundreds of thousands more claimants would have taken further steps to challenge the results if the system was less stressful and more accessible.

In October 2020, the much-delayed tribunal takes place by telephone, following two previous attempts postponed because DWP failed to pass the correct paperwork to the tribunal. Without Dave saying a word, and based just on the medical information before them, the panel awards James Oliver the enhanced daily living component of PIP. A decision on the mobility component must wait, as DWP has again not provided the relevant information. A week or so later, Dave hears James has been awarded the standard rate of mobility. The judge is scathing about DWP's non-participation and the delays it has caused.

In a Facebook post, Dave says: 'Jamie had always wanted the PIP to go towards his funeral costs so his family weren't covering this. He also wanted help with food and energy costs in his final months. It's too late for that as the DWP were content for him to live in a cold, damp, dark, dirty pigsty. But let's hope this is another judgement against the DWP which leads to much-needed change.'

'This was about a government department who thinks it is right to treat the sick, disabled and dying like they just don't have a right to exist. About private assessment companies who employ people where they are essentially paid to lie. About government ministers who haven't got the faintest idea about what it's like to be sick, vulnerable and cast aside like domestic waste.'

22
Philippa Day's Inquest and the 28 'Problems'

The history of DWP, and its role in the countless deaths of disabled benefit claimants, must now return to the Nottingham bedroom of Pip Day, who is soon to become another tragic symbol of the harm caused by the department's decades of slow violence.

When she stumbles into the bedroom, Imogen sees her sister's limbs are spread in unnatural positions across her bed. There is a large bruise in the middle of Pip's forehead, and a bleeding wound. She appears to have had a seizure and hit her head on the bedside table. There is a half-eaten Chinese takeaway on the bed next to her mobile phone, two empty insulin pens, and Netflix is open on her laptop. She is unconscious. The letter from Capita – refusing Pip a home assessment – is lying beside her head on the pillow.

A Word document has been left open but unsaved on Pip's laptop.

> … I thought it was so simple. No drink and take your meds… I need to save my son from this. I need him to feel love and warmth. All I ever wanted was a family somewhere I felt safe, sadly that wasn't meant to be and now I hope my son gets all the love.
>
> My dad. You're the only man I ever loved. Thanks for Tessa for trying. Some people just aren't saveable.

Imogen shouts to her dad to call an ambulance. The call handler tells Imogen to clear the vomit from her sister's mouth and lie her on her side. When the paramedics arrive minutes later, Imogen watches them fight unsuccessfully to find a vein to inject glucose into Pip's blood.

Pip is rushed by ambulance to Queen's Medical Centre. Tests show extensive brain damage. Her brain stem is still functioning, but she is in a coma from which she is unlikely to wake.

While Pip is lying in hospital, Capita – which has been informed she is in a coma – tells the family that if she fails to attend the assessment on 16 August, eight days later, her benefit claim will be cancelled. On 9 September, DWP suddenly deposits £4,000 of benefit arrears in Pip's account, after deciding she is eligible for the enhanced level of both the daily living and mobility components of personal independence payment.

Jane, Pip's mum and a retired nurse, spends 66 of the 69 days her daughter spends in a coma at her bedside. Eventually, Pip's condition deteriorates; there are distressing seizures. The family decide to withdraw all care, apart from pain medication. She dies several days later, on 16 October 2019, with her mother at her bedside.

Imogen will say later that she was 'very angry' at how her sister had been treated. 'We had done what we could as a family to keep her healthy, happy and safe, and an outside agency, never mind a government agency, had interrupted that process,' she would tell the *Dispatches* documentary. Her parents, though, were sad and confused. 'It was almost like they couldn't believe that that was a factor, that this process was so traumatic and poorly designed that it was able to have that impact on disabled people.'

Imogen researches many of the deaths linked to DWP, including those of Faiza Ahmed, Jodey Whiting, and Michael O'Sullivan. She soon realises DWP and its contractors are guilty of systemic failings.

She knows DWP will not admit responsibility. At the start of the inquest process, her parents say there is no need for a lawyer because DWP will be 'open and honest and clear' about any mistakes. But at the first pre-inquest hearing, with Imogen representing the family, she witnesses the 'incredibly aggressive and abrupt' DWP barrister and feels 'incredibly out of my depth.' She is now certain they need legal representation, and approaches Leigh Day, which already represents Jodey Whiting's family.

In November 2020, a hearing examines whether the inquest should look at the wider circumstances of Pip's death. Both DWP and Capita argue against such a finding, but the coroner rules that there should be a wide-ranging inquest.

Imogen tells me the family are determined to fight for an end to the outsourcing of assessments, an overhaul of DWP policies and practices, and for those responsible for Pip's death to be held accountable. 'It's a systemic issue that is killing disabled, vulnerable people on a very regular basis,' she says. 'We need her son to know that we fought for his mother.'

The nine-day inquest begins in Nottingham in the second week of January 2021, 15 months after Pip's death. Pip's parents and her sister give their evidence virtually from their homes in Nottingham and Leeds.

Gordon Clow, assistant coroner for Nottingham and Nottinghamshire, is calm, methodical, compassionate. With the backing of Pip's family, I ask him to release a draft version of the internal process review of Pip's death. DWP has been fighting since August 2014 to prevent the release of the scores of reviews carried out following claimant deaths, and it opposes my request.

No unredacted internal process review (IPR) has ever been released, or even shared with relatives. I argue that Pip's should be released 'in the interests of transparency and accountability' and that this is important because it relates to whether DWP is 'causing or contributing' to the claimant deaths. I say the draft IPR is an 'important historical document that will help to cast a light' on welfare reform.

Simon Hilton, representing DWP, suggests – mistakenly – that I would be able to secure the document through the Freedom of Information Act, which I have used to secure other IPRs. I tell Clow this is untrue, because DWP continues to prevent the release of all but the recommendations of anonymised IPRs. Hilton says he may have misunderstood his instructions from DWP, and tells me: 'This is not some kind of cover-up, which is what you appeared to be implying earlier.'

Sam Jacobs, the Day family's barrister, tells the coroner: 'It is the family's strong view that these documents should be disclosed in the interests of accountability and transparency.'

It is arguable, Clow concludes, that the state has breached its duty to protect the lives of its citizens and to reduce the risk of Pip taking her own life. 'These are important matters,' he says, 'and they therefore weigh in favour of the press being assisted in exercising the right to freedom of expression.' He rules the document should be released.

The draft IPR reveals at least six serious errors were made by at least three DWP civil servants. All appear to have contributed to Pip's decision to take her own life.

On 27 January, Gordon Clow concludes that flaws in the disability benefits system were 'the predominant factor and the only acute factor' that led to Pip taking her own life. He highlights 28 separate 'problems' with the administration of the system that helped cause her death.

It takes the coroner more than two hours to read out his findings, and he ends by telling DWP and Capita he has decided to issue them with prevention of future deaths reports, which will force them to consider changes to the PIP system. DWP will now need to examine the mental health training given to its call handlers and its record-keeping, while Capita must examine the process for changing PIP assessments and ensure letters about this do not create 'unnecessary distress'.

Clow dismisses suggestions made by DWP and Capita that only a few individual errors were made. He says there were significant, systemic flaws.

Among the 28 issues he highlights are the repeated failure to record on her file that Pip needed additional support; and the mistaken decision to remove her benefits after DWP concluded wrongly that she had no 'good cause' for failing to return her claim form in January 2019. He also points to the failure to respond to her mental distress in her call to a DWP telephone agent, and the 'institutional reluctance' to accept evidence from her community psychiatric nurse over the telephone. The 28th problem is Capita's recurring failure to accept that 'requiring a face-to-face assessment at a clinic placed Philippa's safety at risk'.

The coroner concludes that there are 'deficiencies in the system's ability to process PIP claims without causing unnecessary distress to claimants'. Clow does not reach a verdict of suicide, concluding instead that he could 'not be satisfied that it was more likely than not that Philippa intended her death'. But he is 'satisfied on balance of probabilities that Philippa intended to harm herself and to put her life in danger'.

Imogen is 'really happy' with the coroner's conclusions, and praises his 'very full and thorough investigation'. She will continue to campaign for change, and justice for her sister.

Leigh Day's Merry Varney tells me the example set by the coroner and his 'willingness' to investigate the role of DWP 'should be very powerful messages for other coroners'.

In May 2023, a safeguarding review commissioned by agencies in Nottingham – which has been delayed by legal action and the pandemic – concludes that the actions of DWP and Capita had a 'profound' impact on Pip, and that the flawed process 'magnified' her anxiety and 'significantly increased her episodes of self-harm and the risk of suicide'.[1]

DWP tells the review it has worked to build 'a culture of care and compassion' by strengthening its 'vulnerable customer champions' role and introducing 'advanced customer support senior leaders' to provide ways to escalate cases where claimants need 'advanced support'. It claims it has improved how its staff gather evidence for PIP claims, has ensured its records are now permanently 'water-marked' for claimants who need additional support, and now takes extra steps if a claimant fails to respond during a PIP application.

Capita agrees to compensate the family, a sum certain to be in six figures. They had wanted an acknowledgement of wrongdoing, some kind of justice, and financial security for Pip's son. The terms include an agreement to withdraw their legal claim against DWP. Capita will also meet the Days to discuss changes it has made since Pip's death.

Imogen insists she will keep pushing for a public inquiry into the many deaths linked to DWP. 'It's not justice,' she tells me, 'but it is a measure of accountability, a measure of financial accountability, for the mistakes that were made and the trauma we suffered as a result.'

Pip is buried in Thurgarton churchyard, a few miles outside Nottingham. It's a beautiful memorial, says Jane. She is now convinced the reason her daughter took her own life was 'the way she was demeaned and humiliated' by DWP. It made her feel worthless and 'so ill and so fractured that I don't think she could have taken any more', she will tell the *Dispatches* documentary.

'It can be a song, it can be an item of clothing, it can be something her lovely son says. It can be a picture, a movement, the garden. I can see her everywhere; I can feel her everywhere. But I think we're a very strong, together family and we've supported each other incredibly well. But it'll never be the same without Philippa because we're … we're fractured.'

23
The Death of Errol Graham

Dear Sir/Madam

I've had to put in writing how I feel as I find it hard to express myself. I wish I could feel and function normally like anyone else but I find this very hard.

I can't say I have a typical day because some are good, not many, clouded by very bad days. I get up as late as I can so that the day doesn't seem too long. On a good day I open my curtains, but mostly they stay shut.

I find it hard to leave the house on bad days. I don't want to see anyone or talk to anyone. It's not nice living this way.

I'm afraid to put my heating on and sit with a quilt around me to keep me warm. I dread any mail coming, frightened of what it might be because I don't have the means to pay and this is very distressing. Most days I go to bed hungry and I feel I'm not even surviving how I should be. Little things that people brush off are big things to me.

I have come on my own today because I have been unable to share how I feel with anyone because I don't think they would understand. It has made me ill to come here today. It is a big ordeal for me.

My nerves are terrible and coping with this lifestyle wears me out. Sometimes I can't stand to even hear the washing machine and I wish I knew why …

Please judge me fairly. I am a good person but overshadowed by depression. All I want in life is to live normally. That would be the answer to my prayers.

Thank you to all for taking the time to read this letter. I really appreciate it. I don't know how I'll cope when I see you all. I hope I will be OK.

June 2018. The curtains are drawn. There is only one lightbulb in the flat, in the hallway. There is a pile of unopened mail. All the electrical equipment in the flat has been unplugged. The television has been smashed and left in the hallway. In the front bedroom, there are cardboard boxes, piles of letters, some of them left unopened, but it is tidy, organised. On a glass coffee table is the lid of a shoebox. On the lid is a pair of pliers and two large molars.

CDs are scattered across the floor of the living room. The cables from the speakers that had been linked up to the CD player have been cut and are hanging from the door-frame. In the kitchen, there is no food except two tins of tuna, dated 2013. The fridge is empty. Two of the cabinet doors are hanging off their hinges. In the other bedroom, there is a bucket by the bed and a kitchen knife on the floor. There are three mobile phones under the bed, but the batteries have been switched, so none of them fit. The three sim cards have been taped together and jammed into one of the phones and then taped to the phone. Piles of coins have been wrapped in layers of masking tape.

Errol Graham's body is on the floor, as if he has fallen from the bed. The quilt is half on the floor. The bones on his face are protruding, his eyes sunken. His daughter-in-law, Alison Burton, who later identifies his body, would say she had never seen anyone so thin. 'It was beyond anything you can imagine,' she would say. 'He looked so small, like a child. There was nothing left of him.' He is 57 years old and weighs four-and-a-half stone.

* * *

Errol had met Diana at one of the Blues parties that would take place on Friday and Saturday nights around the flats in Radford Road, Nottingham. He loved football, played for the county when he was younger, but supported Liverpool.

They have a son together, but Diana ends the relationship when Lee is about nine months old. 'Errol was a hard person to live with,' she says. She thinks his fears about socialising, and strangers, caused him paralysing anxieties. He would tell her she couldn't go into town with a friend and would allow her just 30 minutes if she wanted to visit someone for tea. 'I used to like nightclubs and going out,' she says, 'but he would just sit at home.'

When she breaks up with Errol, he tells her: 'You don't know what it's like. I feel like jumping out of the window.' They remain close friends, but Diana remembers him being unable to deal with any stress. She leaves him for half an hour with his six-year-old son and when Lee begins to cry, Errol can't cope.

Alison remembers Errol as a quiet, kind and gentle man. 'He would help anybody out. He'd give anybody his last five pounds.' But he is deeply private, and never speaks about the rest of his family, even to Lee. Errol's mum had moved to the US, dying in a car accident. 'He would always listen to your problems, but he'd never burden you with his,' says Alison.

Errol looked after his dad, who lived with significant mental distress. They each had council flats in the same building. Errol, who had previously worked in a warehouse, was first prescribed anti-depressants in 2003, and soon began to claim incapacity benefit due to depression and anxiety. When his dad dies in 2005, Errol finds it hard to cope. A Rastafarian, he cuts off his dreadlocks in the traditional way of expressing his grief. The following year, he tries to take his own life. His doctor describes him as 'a loner' who is reluctant to engage with services. He also has hypothyroidism, which needs to be treated with radioactive iodine. He does not cope well with the deaths of those close to him. 'That seemed to be a trigger point for him,' says Alison.

When the flats where he and his dad had lived are demolished in 2009, Errol moves to a 15th-floor flat in Pine View, a new block across the road from Diana, but is distraught at losing the link with his dad.

Errol and Lee are close. They play football together; they have a shared love of bikes and cycle around Nottingham and the surrounding countryside. Errol spends what little money he has on his prized black Mongoose mountain bike, building it up from just a frame. He loves his music, mostly reggae, and he has a Sky subscription so he can watch football. He doesn't drink, doesn't visit pubs, clubs, or the cinema.

When Lee and Alison have a child of their own, Leelee, in August 2009, Errol will cycle to see them three or four times a week, even though they live 20 miles away. He dotes on Leelee and Alison's daughter Millie. Although he is on benefits, he always buys them gifts on their birthdays and at Christmas.

He will occasionally ask Lee and Alison for some help if money is running low while he waits for his next benefit payment, but it makes him uncomfortable. 'If he said he couldn't come round, we accepted it,' Alison would say later. 'He had his up days and his down days, but he was never aggressive.' He was stubborn, though. If he and Lee argue, it is Lee who must make things right.

Errol sometimes stays the night on Christmas Eve so he can see the children on Christmas morning. Millie is diagnosed as autistic when she is four, and Leelee is also disabled, and their grandad's visits become an important part of their routine. He also sees his grandchildren when they visit Diana. From his flat, he can see through the trees to her front door on Hartley Road, and he will often appear at her back door minutes after they arrive.

In 2011, Errol is assessed for the new employment and support allowance (ESA), as part of the DWP reassessment programme. At some point his benefits are stopped but he is later found not fit for work after an assessment in which he speaks of suicidal thoughts and an attempt to take his own life. In 2013, he is assessed again, and is again found not fit for work, but is told he will be reassessed the following year.

When he has problems with his benefits, Diana will make some calls, lend him a few pounds, or give him some food. Lee and Alison do the same. Errol also uses a local foodbank. At some point, he applies for personal independence payment, but his claim is rejected, and he tells Lee and Alison it would be too stressful to appeal.

The following summer, he is assessed again. By now, there is a 'mental health flag' on the DWP system to alert whoever deals with his claim. His ESA questionnaire is filled in by an advice worker at the community centre. It describes his 'lack of motivation' and how he 'takes a long time to get simple things done'. DWP is told: 'Cannot cope with unexpected changes, upsets my life completely, feel under threat and upset.' And: 'Keep myself to myself, do not engage with strangers, have no social life, feel anxiety and panic in new situations.' He avoids other people because he is likely to 'kick off' and his tendency is to become 'aggressive and abusive'. 'I cannot deal with being challenged in any way and overact,' he tells the advice worker. To avoid this happening, he stays in his flat.

He is assessed by a doctor on 1 June 2014. The doctor says Errol looks 'mentally/psychologically unwell' and 'unkempt'. Although Errol's speech is 'coherent', he notes his 'poor eye contact' and 'poor rapport' and how he appears 'tense' and 'emotional' and describes 'active suicidal thoughts', 'very low mood', and 'daily auditory hallucinations'. He says Errol attempted to take his own life five or six years previously, and is 'hearing voices in his head all the time' which tell him to 'look at the window' or 'clean the door'. He tells the doctor that sometimes he sees moving lights.

He describes how he will usually not get up until after noon, and will visit the shops twice a week, but needs to 'pick himself up' before he can do that and avoids talking to any friends he sees. He claims he has not seen Lee or his grandchildren for 'many months', although the evidence from Lee, Alison, and Diana suggests he is exaggerating or confused. He is again placed in the ESA support group.

It is in the spring of 2015 when things begin to deteriorate. In April, Errol visits the GP surgery and starts behaving aggressively because he cannot get an appointment. A close friend – who he used to play football with – has died, and it has triggered another mental health crisis.

The following month, Errol texts his son to say he has some things he needs to sort out and will not be able to visit for a few days. Diana notices a significant change. He forgets he has visited her and cannot remember which of his friends and family have died.

On 1 June, Diana calls Lee to say his dad is acting strangely. When Lee and Alison walk down the alleyway to the garden, Errol is standing at the back door of Diana's home. 'I had never seen him like that,' Alison says later. 'His pupils had opened up so much. They consumed his eyes.' All he will say is 'Are you OK? Are you OK?' and 'Lee will be all right with you. Lee will be all right with you.' Lee and Alison try to lead him to the car, but he refuses to leave the garden. Then he lashes out. Two of Lee's step-brothers, Diana's sons, come running out to restrain him. They call an ambulance but it takes several police officers to remove him. The ambulance takes him to Highbury Hospital, where there is a mental health unit. Alison is 'in shock'. 'I was really scared for Errol,' she says.

Errol is assessed as lacking capacity to make decisions, so Lee is asked to agree to his dad being sectioned. The next day, Errol is still delusional and keeps telling Lee and Alison that people are out to get him. He is terrified. He tries to block Lee and Alison from going to the patients' courtyard for a cigarette. 'People are trying to kill you out there,' he says. 'They want to kill my family, they want to hurt me.' He begs them to take him home. He tries to hold the door shut when it is time for them to leave.

Lee and Alison continue to visit him nearly every day. They learn that Errol has previously spoken of suicide, has told a friend he will throw himself from his flat, and has heard voices telling him to jump.

His consultant psychiatrist concludes that Errol has experienced an 'adjustment disorder' due to 'psychosocial stressors compounded by cannabis use' and that there are no convincing hallucinations or delusions that suggest a more serious long-term mental health condition.

From 8 June, the hospital allows Errol short periods of escorted and unescorted leave. Lee and Alison feel it is too early for him to leave Highbury, and that he is not as well as he pretends to be. They arrange to pick Errol up for a short period of leave, and take him back later that day.

On 13 June, Alison arrives at Highbury alone, as Lee is ill. Errol arrives at reception with a couple of near-empty bin-liners. He says he wants to do some laundry. She takes him to withdraw money from a cashpoint and then to his flat. She waits in the car while he puts his clothes in the washing machine. When he fails to reappear, Alison tries calling him. The second time she calls, he answers the phone. 'I am not coming out,' he tells her. 'I am not going back. I want to be at home.'

Alison drives home to fetch Lee. When they return, Errol won't let them in. He shouts through the letterbox: 'I am not going back to hospital. I just want to be in my flat.' Police officers arrive early the next morning, but leave without him. The hospital applies for a warrant to return him to the ward, but it is rejected by a magistrate. Three days later, a member of the mental health crisis team visits Errol and raises no immediate concerns.

Eight days later, the Highbury psychiatrist visits Errol at the home of his friend Liz. He reports no psychotic symptoms and concludes he is not acutely unwell. Errol makes it clear he does not want to return to hospital and wants to stop some of his medication as it is making him sleepy. The psychiatrist concludes that Errol has capacity to make these decisions.

On 9 July, Errol sees the crisis team again. They again report no psychotic symptoms, suicidal thoughts, or anything else of concern. Errol tells them he has stopped taking all his mental health medication. They conclude again that he has capacity to make this decision, although they ask the psychiatrist for advice. Although Errol does not want his family to know he wants to be discharged, the psychiatrist tells Lee about this decision. Errol is discharged from his inpatient stay and from the mental health crisis team. There are no subsequent follow-ups from mental health services in the next month.

Lee and Alison keep ringing and 'pestering' the hospital but they fail to persuade Highbury and mental health services to re-engage with Errol.

Meanwhile, Alison, Lee, and Diana are taking Errol food they cook at Diana's house across the road. They wait until they hear a sound or see him through the letterbox, and then tell him they are leaving it outside the door. On one occasion, he opens the door slightly and accepts some money.

Liz tells Lee and Alison that Errol is keeping in touch with her and seeing other people they know, so they stop taking the food. Errol is furious that they allowed him to be sectioned. They take a step back. 'The last thing we wanted to do was be responsible for him not coming out of the flat,' Alison says later. 'He was deliberately keeping away from us and whenever we were around, he would not leave his flat. Whereas when we weren't there, he was going out and getting food. He had a mental health support worker, and we thought our involvement wasn't going to help.'

They soon begin to worry again, as Errol is seeing less of Liz. In July 2015, Lee and Alison see Errol on his bike as they are leaving Diana's house. They shout to Errol, but he looks straight through them. They visit him, but he won't open his door. Lee shouts through the letterbox: 'I will leave you alone, but I just want to know you are alright.' There is no answer.

On 23 August, Liz calls the crisis team and says Errol's behaviour is again causing her concern. It is possible that the mental health trust sends Errol's GP a fax, but subsequently neither the trust nor the surgery can produce it.

'We just didn't know what to do,' says Alison. 'We didn't want to keep pressing him and going to his door; we were worried that would send him over the edge. We felt that it was safest for him for us to stay away.'

They receive regular reports that Errol is being seen at the nearby Aldi and has been seen out in Radford. But there are reports of him shouting at people, and he smashes up displays in a local shop. Other than this, there is no indication that he is as ill as the night he was sectioned. They ask Liz, Diana, and other friends to tell Errol their door is always open.

Lee has psoriasis, and the stress has left his skin raw and bleeding. He has been left deeply hurt. Alison's dad has had a heart attack, and her health has also been affected by the stress. She has several long-term health conditions, including fibromyalgia, hypermobility syndrome, Raynaud's syndrome, and bronchial asthma, which all flare up when under stress. She also has cysts on her bones and muscles. The pain has worsened. She has to quit her job as a hospital cook.

In August 2016, the anxiety and stress caused by being locked out of his dad's life, and the guilt he feels at having him sectioned, contribute to Lee's involvement in an argument that leads to a fight. It was out of character, says Alison. 'He's not the sort of person who would randomly engage in a fight. He's normally the person to try and talk people down. It was a reaction from Lee I've never seen before.' The argument starts over the phone, and Lee tries to 'calm the situation', but she says he loses control when the other man threatens their children. It is a serious assault, and he has never tried to excuse his actions. He is bailed for nine months, and the following May is found guilty and jailed for eight years for grievous bodily harm. While on bail he tries to see his dad, visiting him every day. He shouts through the letterbox, telling his dad he is sorry, asking him to forgive him.

Lee will later tell the *Dispatches* documentary: 'My cousins used to go round as well, knock on his door and shout through the letterbox. I couldn't really force myself onto him, because you can push someone into a corner, can't you, and they could end up doing something stupid, so you had to give him that space. But we tried, obviously, as much as we could to help him.'

Alison is now trying to cope with her own health problems while Lee is in prison, and is looking after her two disabled children. 'I was barely managing to keep everything together,' she says, 'so I didn't keep trying to reach out to Errol. I assumed he was getting on with his life as normal, that he was still angry with us but that he knew our door remained open.'

Errol continues to visit Diana through 2015 and into 2016, although he never comes inside the house. He stands at the back garden gate and talks to her. One of the last times Diana sees him, she and a friend are in the centre of Nottingham, about to go on a coach trip. Errol is at the coach station with his bike. He starts shouting at her. 'You said you would be there for me. Where are you? Don't go. Don't go.' He starts shouting at the traffic.

The following year, in the autumn of 2017, Liz's mum dies, and Errol reacts badly at the funeral. Liz shouts at Errol. It is the last time she sees him.

Meanwhile, failings at Errol's GP surgery mean he is not recalled for check-ups or blood tests for his depression or hypothyroidism.

Errol does not book further appointments, perhaps ashamed of his behaviour at the surgery in the spring of 2015.

In June 2017, DWP asks Errol's GP to complete an ESA113 form. The GP notes on the form that Errol has not been seen by a GP since 2013. Because there was no up-to-date ESA50 questionnaire, a Maximus nurse decides he will need a face-to-face assessment. He is sent an appointment for 31 August. He does not turn up. Maximus writes to ask why. The form is not returned. On 9 October, a DWP decision-maker calls him and sends a text, but he fails to answer. They call again the next day. Again, there is no response.

DWP orders a safeguarding visit because of a mental health flag against his name on its system. The referral states: 'Available medical evidence includes depression. The available evidence therefore suggests vulnerability and justifies a safeguarding visit.' Two visits are made to Errol's block of flats, on 16 and 17 October, but on each occasion no contact with Errol is made, and a letter is left. He fails to respond to the letters.

On 17 October, DWP concludes that 'because he has not proved good cause for his failure to attend, he is treated as having capability for work.' DWP sends him a letter telling him his ESA will end, which could also affect his housing benefit. That stops, too. His gas is cut off in October, because Nottingham City Homes, which runs the council's housing stock, has been unable to gain access for a safety check. Although he has an electric cooker, there is no hot water and no central heating throughout the winter.

It is not clear whether he opens the DWP letters or sees the text message. Alison says his trust in DWP had been damaged when at a previous assessment his claim was rejected because he had ironed his clothes to attend the face-to-face meeting. 'From that point on, he was scared that every time you go to an assessment you could lose everything.'

At this point, DWP has no information about Errol dated post-2014. His ESA85A* form from 2013 states that he had suicidal thoughts and there is 'likely to be a risk to his own physical or mental

* The ESA85A is a medical report form completed by the assessor if the claimant has not had a face-to-face assessment.

health if he was not found to be of limited capability to work'. The DWP decision-maker has access to this form. No attempt is made to contact any healthcare or other professionals involved in his case. As a coroner will later conclude, DWP has no idea whether withdrawing his benefits will put his life at risk.

Errol's rent arrears and other debts begin to build up. In February 2018, a manager from Nottingham City Homes (NCH) speaks to Errol through his front door. Twice Errol shouts: 'What do you want?' and he punches the door. The manager later tries to phone both Errol and Lee, but both numbers are disconnected. Although Errol recorded on his housing application in 2010 that he has depression, NCH staff are unaware of his mental health condition. For the next four months, he fails to respond to letters and visits from NCH.

Nothing else is known about what happens to Errol during 2017 and 2018. He has no money, and he faces the threat of eviction. He does not ask his family or anyone else for help.

On the morning of 20 June 2018, bailiffs knock on Errol's front door to evict him. There is no answer. They force their way into the flat. They find his body lying on the floor of his bedroom.

It is Alison and Diana who identify Errol's body at Queen's Medical Centre. 'I remember walking in and seeing his face,' Alison will say later. 'I couldn't speak.' Diana has to say the words: 'Yes, that is him.'

'Errol's body was cold,' Alison told me. 'He had a white sheet covered up to his neck. He was so thin. I touched his arm and it felt like there was no fat there at all. His face was so drawn. He looked like he had aged 50 years. Practically every bone in his face was protruding. His eyes were sunken. His hairline was a lot further back than I remembered… There was nothing left of him.'

They are both in tears. Alison is struggling to catch her breath. Afterwards, she can't get the image out of her head. She receives the keys for Errol's flat but has only 48 hours to clear it. In one of the rooms, she finds a shoebox lid, a pair of heavy-duty pliers, and 'a couple of back molar teeth with huge roots'. 'I looked at it and realised that Errol must have pulled out his own teeth,' she says. 'When I found those teeth, I felt ill, it made me feel sick. I couldn't imagine how much pain Errol must have been in to resort to ripping his molar teeth out.'

Alison's mum is with her, and they find a letter Errol had written to the Maximus assessors but never handed over.

> I'm afraid to put my heating on and sit with a quilt around me to keep me warm. I dread any mail coming, frightened of what it might be because I don't have the means to pay and this is very distressing. Most days I go to bed hungry and I feel I'm not even surviving how I should be … Please judge me fairly. I am a good person but overshadowed by depression. All I want in life is to live normally …

Alison says it broke her heart to read the letter. 'Errol was never able to share how he truly felt with me and Lee. This letter was the first and only time we got close to Errol's daily struggles.'

Lee is allowed to attend the funeral, cuffed at the waist so he can help carry his dad's coffin. About 300 people attend. Millie reads a poem, and she finishes by saying: 'We love you grandad and we will miss you always.' A group of Errol's friends, including some of his old football mates, pay for the reception. There are photographs of Errol in picture frames on a table, and Alison tells mourners to take a photograph to remember him. By the end, only one is left.

* * *

In October 2018, research by academics at the University of Essex, and Inclusion London,[1] concludes that the system of sanctions and conditions imposed on disabled people placed in the ESA work-related activity group (WRAG) – who can see their benefits cut for weeks if they fail to carry out certain activities to their jobcentre adviser's satisfaction – has a 'significantly detrimental' effect on their mental health. The researchers say this approach is 'psychologically toxic', intellectually 'incoherent', counter-productive and 'arbitrary', and that it causes 'a state of almost constant anxiety'.

In May 2019, DWP finally admits that the prevention of future deaths reports written by coroners after the deaths of Stephen Carré and Michael O'Sullivan, and a series of peer reviews into the deaths of ESA claimants, were not shared with the team that reviewed the work capability assessment.

A summary of the information commissioner's discussions with DWP – following a complaint I had made against the department – proves neither the peer reviews nor the coroners' letters were sent to Paul Litchfield. DWP had contacted those members of Litchfield's team still working for the department and asked them to search electronic and paper records. I am told: 'Consultation with the ex-review team elicited statements that no such information was received from DWP nor were any physical files sent to stores.'

DWP's excuse is that Litchfield never asked for the reports. But a DWP spokesperson is unable to explain how Litchfield's team could have requested the peer reviews and coroners' letters if they did not know they existed. Two years later, Litchfield will confirm, in evidence to the work and pensions select committee, that DWP failed to show him these documents.[2]

* * *

Errol Graham's inquest takes place in June 2019, and among those giving evidence are Alison, Errol's psychiatrist and community psychiatric nurse, his GP, the police officer who attended Errol's flat after his body was discovered – PC Emily Dunn – who Alison says was 'absolutely fantastic' in the following months, and Alison Hunt and David Carew from DWP.

The two senior DWP civil servants would not have had to give evidence if Alison had not contacted the coroner with her concerns. She says the 'anger kicked in' as she started to piece together what had happened from Errol's papers. She sent hundreds of emails to the coroner's office as she uncovered new facts. The coroner helped the family obtain paperwork the authorities were refusing to release for 'data protection' reasons.

'We felt like we didn't exist, we were nobody's concern,' says Alison. 'I was asking, "How does this happen? How can the system do this to him?"' She decides she is not going to let DWP get away with the way it treated Errol. 'I've always been a very stubborn person,' she says. 'I don't like people thinking that because they have a badge or because they are in a position of power, that entitles them to step on people like they're nothing.'

Alison and her family cannot afford a lawyer to represent them at the inquest, but DWP pays for a leading barrister to defend its failures.

DWP tells the inquest that because Errol had not seen his GP since 2013, and there was no recent ESA questionnaire, he had been asked to attend a WCA. But the inquest also hears that he had not been asked to complete an ESA questionnaire, even though he had previously completed and returned them – with assistance – for previous claims.

Although DWP has produced forms from his earlier assessments, the documents from his 2014 WCA are not in the inquest bundle. They would have shown exactly how ill Errol was just three years before the department suddenly stopped his benefits. Alison Hunt, DWP's manager for legacy benefit delivery in central England, says those documents 'would have been very much like the last one' in 2013. This is not accurate. The reports from his face-to-face assessment would have shown Errol's 'active suicidal thoughts' and that he was 'hearing voices in his head all the time'.

Hunt says the department carried out two safeguarding visits because Errol was 'classed as a vulnerable person' and they 'wouldn't want to stop the money without being 100 per cent sure that he understood what he was doing by not attending'. When asked why his money was stopped without getting this assurance, she says DWP 'had no indicators that anything was wrong' and did 'the maximum that we could do to try to get hold of Mr Graham before we stopped his money'.

Asked if it was a reasonable decision to make, she says: 'I think at the time, with what we had, yes, it was unfortunately, very sad, but the right decision for us to have made.'

A psychiatrist tells the inquest that Errol had been vulnerable to 'life stressors' and it was likely that the loss of income when his benefits were stopped was the final, devastating stressor that pushed him over the edge.

Assistant coroner Dr Elizabeth Didcock concludes that the 'safety net that should surround vulnerable people like Errol in our society had holes within it'. She criticises DWP directly. 'He needed the DWP to obtain more evidence [from his GP] at the time his ESA was stopped, to make a more informed decision about him, particularly following the failed safeguarding visits.' But she decides not to write a prevention of future deaths report because DWP insists it is already reviewing its safeguarding. She is convinced by DWP's promises, which evidence will later show were deeply misleading.

Didcock insists that DWP's commitment 'must be converted into robust policy and guidance for DWP staff' and it must ensure that 'all evidence that can reasonably be gathered is put together about a client, before a benefit is ceased'. She becomes the latest coroner to demand that DWP acts on the issue of further medical evidence, and the latest to be ignored by the department. She concludes that Errol died from starvation.

After Alison contacts me about Errol's death six months later, I ask Didcock if she is aware of the many previous deaths – including two reported by coroners – that have been linked to similar DWP failings, including the failure to secure further medical evidence. She tells me she does not have the legal powers to reopen the inquest, but will ask DWP what has happened to its safeguarding review. I later obtain evidence through a freedom of information request that shows David Carew presented misleading evidence to the inquest.

Carew, the department's chief psychologist, had said he was leading the safeguarding review, and that it was set to be completed that autumn, with a report on its findings. 'I leave this building today very clear in my own mind that the work we are involved in in the current time has a degree of urgency about it,' he tells Didcock.

But DWP tells me later that this safeguarding work is instead 'ongoing and will continue as a key part of continuous improvement and learning', that there 'is no formal commission to publish a review', and 'no formal review team'. It adds: 'There is not a final report.'

'DWP showed they were not there with any intention to learn lessons,' Alison Burton tells me. 'I don't know how long they think they are going to keep getting away with it. They think they can keep sweeping it under the carpet. I think the carpet is getting a bit full of crap now.'

In September 2019, just three months after Errol's inquest, work and pensions secretary Amber Rudd secures £106 million from the Treasury to fund what the department calls a DWP Excellence Plan. A third of the money is allocated to improving safety, support for 'customers with complex needs', decision-making, and learning from its mistakes. In all, £66 million is allocated to 'support vulnerable people'.

The department plans to set up what it calls a serious case panel, with 'independent membership', to examine deaths of claimants linked to its actions. It also intends to 'reduce the impact of serious cases (including customer suicide)' and measure the department's success in reducing the number of such cases. It describes how a new 'Safeguarding Improvement Team' will 'proactively introduce processes, procedures and policies to protect vulnerable customers and improve the effectiveness of DWP interventions'.

Staff will be given extra time to respond to signs of 'customer vulnerability', refer claimants to specialist support, and prevent 'an escalation of vulnerability and risk to customer welfare'. One of the 'benefits' will be 'increased effective suicide/harm prevention'. There are also plans for an independent review of the department's sanctions policy.

Rudd appears to have drawn up a serious plan for addressing the department's toxic legacy and the hostile environment that has led to countless deaths of claimants, including Errol's. But just as the funding is agreed by the Treasury, Rudd quits as work and pensions secretary over Brexit. She is replaced by right-winger Dr Thérèse Coffey.

Freedom of information requests, by myself and particularly by a welfare rights expert who prefers to stay anonymous, will later show how DWP abandoned much of the plan under Coffey's leadership.[3]

The plan to pilot a scheme to support claimants who were 'beginning to struggle to cope' was abandoned; so too was the proposal to measure how successful DWP was in reducing the number of 'serious cases'; I was also told there was no such thing as a 'Safeguarding Improvement Team'; and, although the serious case panel was set up, Coffey abandoned plans for its members to be independent – instead, it was filled with senior DWP executives. Plans to measure how often staff were responding to signs of 'customer vulnerability' and how many claimants were referred for 'complex needs' support were also abandoned.

There have been some improvements, Coffey insists in March 2020. DWP decision-makers are now 'empowered' to go back to Atos, Maximus, and Capita to seek more information if any 'gaps or concerns' have been raised by an assessment report. They can also contact the claimant. Local areas now carry out 'case conferencing' on complex cases, often working with other agencies or local organisations, while guidance for staff in dealing with 'customers with complex needs' has been strengthened, as has mental health training for staff. She says DWP has improved the capacity and capability of its IPR team, improved communication with coroners, and now 'rigorously' tracks recommendations from both IPRs and the serious case panel. The department is also recruiting 37 'safeguarding leaders'.

But I later learn that – in addition to abandoning the excellence plan – Coffey has scrapped plans for an independent review of its sanctions policy.[4] DWP blames the pandemic and 'differing priorities' under Coffey's leadership.

* * *

Anne-Marie O'Sullivan has continued to work quietly and with astonishing determination and perseverance to uncover the truth about her father's death, with support from the family's MP Sir Keir Starmer – soon to become the new Labour leader – and welfare rights expert Nick Dilworth. They will later show how DWP made at least 61 errors in dealing with her father's benefit claim.

Anne-Marie tells me that during a General Medical Council (GMC) investigation into the fitness to practise of Dr Fathy Awad Sherif, the orthopaedic surgeon who carried out Michael's face-to-face assessment in March 2013, the doctor's representatives told GMC investigators: 'Following the conversion of Incapacity Benefit to ESA, the DWP put immense pressure on Atos disability analysts to deem claimants fit for work when they previously would have qualified for benefits.' DWP has insisted for years that no such pressure was placed on Atos.

GMC issues a warning to Dr Sherif about his fitness for practise, after finding his WCA report was 'significantly below the standard expected of a reasonably competent Disability Analyst' and that he did 'not meet with the standards required of a doctor' and 'risks bringing the profession into disrepute'.

DWP is restricted in how it can comment because of the 2019 general election campaign, but it claims it sets high standards for assessment providers but does not set targets to find claimants fit for work. It points yet again to its five independent reviews and says it has implemented the vast majority of their recommendations. Improvements include introducing mental health training for all staff dealing directly with claimants, appointing mental health champions to advise assessors, and allowing for further evidence to be requested when considering mandatory reconsiderations.

* * *

I first hear about Errol Graham's death in January 2020, after being contacted by Alison, who by now has been fighting for justice since 2018. It has taken her some months to persuade Lee to allow her to go public with the story of what happened to his father.

When I tell Denise McKenna, from the Mental Health Resistance Network, about Errol's death, she says the network is 'absolutely devastated and saddened beyond words' to hear of the circumstances and 'enraged that the DWP continues to treat the lives of people who live with mental distress as disposable'.

'This level of cruelty is outside of anything that would happen in a civilised society,' she says. 'The government is well aware that the social security system is causing deaths. There should be a criminal investigation into Mr Graham's death. We can no longer say that such deaths are accidental or due to some error. This is deliberate and therefore goes beyond manslaughter.'

There is a huge public and media reaction to the three stories I publish on the DNS website on 20 January 2020. I put Alison and the family in touch with Leigh Day, the solicitors who are working with Jodey Whiting's family.

Asked by Labour's Debbie Abrahams about the case the following week, Justin Tomlinson, the minister for disabled people, expresses no sympathy with the family, regret or condolences, instead using time-honoured DWP techniques to obscure the truth. 'I thank the honourable lady for that question,' he says. 'She has been a long-standing campaigner against Labour's work capability assessment, introduced in 2008. We agree: that is why we commissioned five independent reviews and implemented more than 100 recommendations. Working with the Royal College of Psychiatrists, we are making sure that our frontline staff are fully trained to be in the best place to identify people at risk of suicide.'

Alison says she would like to see a criminal investigation into the actions of Iain Duncan Smith, Chris Grayling, and senior DWP civil servants. 'It's down to them why this happened in the first place,' she says. 'Despite being told repeatedly, they continue to allow it to happen.'

Duncan Smith has just received a knighthood, and Alison tells me: 'What kind of message does that give? You're basically saying to the families who are victims of the system that their lives do not matter. He may as well knock on my front door and kick me in the face.'

Just two weeks later, the National Audit Office (NAO) reveals persistent and serious flaws in DWP's internal process review (IPR) system.[5] Astonishingly, the department has told the NAO there is 'no tracking or monitoring of the status' of the recommendations made in its IPRs and so it 'does not know whether the suggested improvements are implemented'.

Three years earlier, DWP had made an almost identical confession to the information commissioner and promised to correct the system, after I had lodged a complaint about its failure to say what action it had taken in response to some of the 49 peer reviews. DWP had admitted then that it kept no records of what happened to the recommendations made by its reviews. Now, three years after insisting that it had 'identified changes to improve accountability and responsibility and ensure that recommendations were identified, logged centrally and followed up so that outcomes were tracked, audited and understood', it appears to be confessing that it lied to the information commissioner.

In July, Alison wins the right to have DWP's safeguarding policies examined by the high court. She wants a declaration that DWP violated Errol's right to life under the Human Rights Act, and that DWP's failure to contact individuals such as relatives, social workers, and GPs to establish if it is safe to stop benefit payments to any claimant in a vulnerable situation is unlawful.

The case is built upon hours of research Alison carried out in the months leading to the inquest. It also relies heavily on evidence I have collected over the last six years while researching other deaths linked to DWP. 'It is important because so many have been let down and families have been torn apart,' she tells me. 'There has been no accountability.'

In September, Thérèse Coffey insists publicly that the department does not have a 'duty of care' and 'does not have any statutory safeguarding responsibilities'. 'I do not think it is the responsibility of DWP to have that statutory care duty,' she says. 'We are not the local councils, the social services, the doctors and other people who have that.'

Alison accuses Coffey of being 'heartless' and disrespecting all the families who have lost relatives because of DWP's actions. 'It's only right and caring that you make sure of a person's safety before you do anything that could kill them,' she says. 'It's common sense.

People like Errol have died because of it, because of the department's lack of care, its lack of concern for people's safety.'

In December, another batch of IPRs obtained under the Freedom of Information Act show again that DWP staff are failing to follow the department's guidance on how to respond to claimants who declare they intend to self-harm or take their own lives. At least five IPRs carried out between 2014 and 2019 following the deaths of claimants recommended that staff should be reminded of the guidance. At least two of the IPRs say the failure to follow the guidance is a 'recurring theme'. One of them is likely to have been completed following the suicide of Faiza Ahmed.

The following March, the high court rejects the claim[6] that DWP acted unlawfully by not making further enquiries about Errol's mental health before it cut off his ESA. It also rejects the claim that DWP's safeguarding policy is unlawful. The court had heard that DWP had changed its policy so its decision-makers must consider contacting a next-of-kin or other agencies, and must hold a case conference, after two failed safeguarding visits to a claimant's home.

The judge says this is 'a significant improvement to the policy'. He describes DWP's actions as 'reasonable' and insists that it 'conducted the inquiries which it considered reasonably necessary to find out whether there was a "good cause" for his failure to attend the assessment, and Mr Graham sadly did not engage at all'.

Alison is 'stunned' by the judgment. 'It's blaming Errol for his own death,' she says.

When the long-awaited safeguarding review into Errol's death is finally published in May 2023,[7] it is critical of DWP, but not damning. I soon discover why. The department had failed to provide the independent reviewer with the documents from Errol's 2014 work capability assessment that would have shown how Errol had been experiencing significant mental distress just three years before his ESA was suddenly withdrawn by the department in October 2017.

Just as it had kept these documents from the inquest into Errol's death, and only released them to the high court days before the judicial review hearing, DWP has deliberately prevented this vital evidence from being considered by a statutory investigation.

When I share the missing documents with the Nottingham City Safeguarding Adults Board, it announces a review. After I tell her what has happened, Debbie Abrahams raises the concerns in an adjournment debate. Tom Pursglove, the minister for disabled people, claims it is 'simply not true' that 'officials hid information from the board'. He blames the safeguarding review for not being clearer in its request for information.

Alison says the department is denying Errol the justice he is entitled to in death. It is still 'pulling dirty little tricks', she says. It is yet another cover-up.

Six months later, the review's author, Sylvia Manson, publishes an addendum to the report. It concludes that DWP should not have stopped Errol's benefits. She is now much more critical of the department. The 2014 report 'should have raised sufficient flags about whether there may have been "good cause" for why [Errol] had not responded to requests for a review and triggered making further enquiries with other agencies', she concludes. DWP's 'deceitful' behaviour is no surprise to Alison. 'If it is committed to improving its services and protecting its claimants, as it claims every time, why be deceitful?' she tells me. 'All it says to me is they have no interest in improving their services.'

Alison has given birth to another son, Lorenzo. Lee is working as a stonemason. He is still finding it difficult to come to terms with what happened to his dad. 'It cuts him deep,' says Alison. 'He's working all the hours, he's working to distract himself.' Some weeks he works 70 hours. He is constantly asking himself if he should have pushed harder to force himself back into his dad's life.

They visit Errol's grave often, and they revealed the gender of the baby earlier that year at the graveside. Millie couldn't handle seeing the grave for a long time, but she now seems to find it a comfort. Lee visits often on his own, to be close once again to his dad.

24

The Death of Roy Curtis

'THIS IS WHEN MY NIGHTMARE BEGAN'. The words are scrawled in red capitals across the top of the letter. It is the covering page of a capability for work questionnaire Roy Curtis had been asked to complete by CHDA, otherwise known as Maximus. The letter is dated 12 December 2016. It is in a folder of letters Roy placed on a shelf under his coffee table.

Detective constable Lucy Jarrett, who finds the folder, will say later: 'The words across the letters were as if the author had been distressed about his situation and that benefits and allowances had been stopped and he had been asking for help from various agencies.'

Another letter from CHDA told him to attend an assessment in Milton Keynes on 15 February 2017. On this one, Roy has written: 'I CAN'T GO TO MKC BECAUSE OF PANIC ATTACKS. I WAS REFUSED A HOME VISIT.' He has the assessment moved to Aylesbury, but he is still denied a home assessment, writing on another letter: 'SO I HAD TO GO FAR AWAY ON A STRESSFUL TRIP.'

The assessment leads to his benefits being cut, and Roy is moved into the work-related activity group, for claimants who must take steps to move into work. He writes on this one: 'I WAS ASSURED I WOULD BE OK. THEN YOU CUT MY FUCKING INCOME???? I ASKED WHY. I HEARD NOTHING.'

There is also an appointment to see a work coach ('I WENT WITH SUPPORT IN EXTREME DISTRESS'), and, crucially, a letter from DWP, dated 18 August 2018, telling Roy his ESA is being stopped because he failed to attend another assessment. 'NO SHIT! I DON'T NEED ONE', he scrawls in red ink. 'I HAVE SAID OVER AND OVER AGAIN I AM UNFIT FOR WORK.'

Within three months, Roy Curtis – previously known as Ayman Habayeb – will have taken his own life. But the truth about why he died and who was responsible is even more disturbing than the scrawled notes he has left behind.

* * *

From a young age, Ayman had difficulties with social interaction. Although he will not be formally diagnosed for nearly 20 years, a speech and language therapy consultation report, written when he is just four, suggests a 'context' of autism. He is 'an attractive little boy … who appeared solemn and uncertain'. He plays alone and 'made no attempt to communicate with other children, though at one stage he briefly joined another child who was playing with a railway'. He 'very much seemed the outsider'.

The report concludes: 'It appears that Ayman has difficulties which extend beyond language, affecting aspects of social development. These centre around relationships, communication, and imagination and suggest that autism is the context in which to consider these difficulties.'

The family – Ayman, his parents, and his younger sister – move to Kuwait, but they return to the UK a few years later following concerns over his 'bizarre' behaviour, and social isolation. He is seen by a psychologist. They move to Dubai. At 17, Ayman attempts suicide.

He moves back to the UK for university, but fails to register or attend any lectures, and when his parents cannot contact him, they request a police welfare check that finds him in his room with, according to a later assessment, 'poor physical health, but no concern for his mental health'.

Ayman will insist he has never really related to his family and is comfortable with this situation, although they struggle to accept this. As a teenager, he has frequently told his family he was never 'wired up for life' and will end his own life by the age of 21.

There are other suicide attempts, and a health assessment in May 2012, when he is nearly 21, following concerns raised by his mother.

He is living in his parents' home in Milton Keynes, while they make frequent trips to visit him from Dubai. He has not been eating – although his parents provide him with money – no longer has a mobile phone, and is underweight.

The two health professionals who assess him find him in his bedroom wearing his pyjamas, with 'disheveled long curly hair and a lot of facial hair'. He explains he is 'happy in his own world' and 'did not like others interfering in his life'. He is 'tearful' but will not admit he might be depressed. There is foil on the windows to stop the sun shining on his computers. He has never been employed and does not feel he 'should have to work or study to be an accepted member of society'. It has been months since he left the house. He wants people to accept that he wants to die.

A few weeks later, Ayman is diagnosed as autistic by the autism assessment and diagnosis service run by the Milton Keynes joint health and social care service. His assessment finds his social approaches 'usually inappropriate, one-sided, and naïve and can be regarded as peculiar'. His intelligence is above average. As a young adult, he had become 'increasingly frustrated and angry with his apparent inability to meet the expectations and requirements for social and vocational independence'. His social care needs will 'continue to be a concern' and remain unmet if he lives alone, with the possibility of self-neglect. The psychologist concludes that Ayman should be 'urgently considered for a supportive living arrangement and receive assistance with his social and vocational needs'. This is eventually provided by Milton Keynes council. Later in the year, Roy (he had changed his name from Ayman Habayeb to Roy Curtis) spends about two weeks in the Campbell Centre, an inpatient mental health unit in Milton Keynes, which may have followed a suicide attempt.

In January 2016, he is judged no longer to need the support he has been receiving and moves into a housing association flat on the edge of town, on the first floor of a smart, new block overlooking the Ashland Lakes parkland. His family will later say that this move – and the council's 'catalogue of failures and misjudgment' – will contribute to his death. But just as important a factor, they believe, is that he has been hounded for years by DWP.

The picture painted by these medical reports is only partially accurate. His friends stress his kindness and generosity, that he had several relationships, and the contributions he made to online communities.

One school friend from Dubai who posted online after his death writes: 'Ayman's character, jokes, wit, genius and love are the reasons why we all celebrated him… I hope we can all share fond memories of him, his quirks, his love, his hugs, his humour, his dancing, his kindness, everything you could wish for in a friend.'

Another school friend writes: 'Advocate for the power of hugs and helping others, bouncing through school with your Free Hugs sign will be how I remember you always. Incredibly loved and incredibly missed.'

Online posts show how he was thoughtful and considerate. One online friend will write later: 'He was always willing and eager to help anyone with problems, technical, personal or otherwise. I keep hearing from other friends how he helped them through tough times or challenges, or even arranged to have a pizza delivered to someone who was hungry or broke.'

His neighbour, Tobias Meakins, writes later of how Roy had collected hundreds of train announcements in English and Welsh for a project. Tobias will often see Roy early in the morning – about 6am – coming downstairs to put his bins out or visit the shop while he is waiting for a lift to work.

Their last interaction comes in late October 2018. Roy has heard that Tobias has been unwell, and he has put together a 'get well soon hamper' with chocolates, tissues, Ribena, and Night Nurse. He messages him, saying the package is outside his flat. At the time, Roy is heavily in debt because of his DWP issues.

He cuts off all contact with his family in around 2013. They spend years trying to find him, with his mother repeatedly contacting the Samaritans, the police, and the council. She never gives up trying to find him, and following his death she spends years campaigning for justice for her son.

His father, Fuad, will speak at his funeral of how his son had been 'conceived and born with love, brought up and grew on love, and now we are giving him back with nothing but love'.

* * *

DWP starts to cast its grim shadow over Roy's life. He is relying on the state for support, and DWP is insisting he attends face-to-face assessments that cause him significant distress. A letter from his partner David is handed over at his work capability assessment in Aylesbury on 3 March 2017.

David has written:

> He is extremely distressed by the assessment process, which exacerbates his conditions, and is causing him significant mental health risks, including suicidal thoughts at the prospect of being found fit for work… Roy is distressed by leaving his flat, and cannot go out without difficulty… I believe that the stress of attending a regular job, or even preparatory work-related activities, would be extremely likely to distress him to such an extent, and to cause his mental health to deteriorate, such that *he would again be at risk of attempting suicide.*

Despite this plea, Roy is told on 7 April his benefits will be cut, and he is placed in the ESA work-related activity group, which means he has to attend meetings and possibly join a work programme to help him prepare for the job market.

A note, likely written after he is told about this decision and probably attached to his request for a mandatory reconsideration, describes his state of mind. 'I want this to be over with,' he writes. 'If it were up to me I would just end my life and not be a burden to the system, but it's not up to me is it???' He adds: 'PLEASE HELP ME. I don't know what else to do. I AM NOT FIT FOR WORK!!!'

His situation only worsens. The following March, he is told to attend another face-to-face assessment. He refuses, and his benefits are removed. He is told of the decision on 15 August, and scrawls on the letter in red ink: 'I HAVE SAID OVER AND OVER AGAIN I AM UNFIT FOR WORK.' He asks for a reconsideration but on 21 September the department rubber-stamps the decision.

It is around this time that Roy writes a statement – a coroner at his inquest will describe it as 'remarkable' – which he posts online. In it, he says he has decided to take his own life, and he even gives a date: Wednesday 19 September 2018. He describes how ESA has been his only income and he is therefore 'no longer able to pay rent or afford to eat', writing: 'I decided that I would not bother fighting this, and will exit instead. I have written this page to clearly explain my decision to friends, and to answer anticipated questions.'

Roy is adamant he will not change his mind. 'If I am not going to be listened to, and if the DWP are not going to understand that my condition is immutable, then I am not going to play along.' He says he cannot fight DWP anymore. 'I am out of energy. I only exist to do what I want to do; dealing with paperwork, making phone calls, and feeling anxious every day about whether I am going to be homeless are things I do not want to do.'

He explains he is unfit for work because he is 'not wired for it'. 'I have Aspergers syndrome, chronic depression, and I am chronically lazy. The thought of getting a job makes me extremely unhappy, to the point where I become suicidal.' He describes how he will end his life, and posts a video showing an attempt to do so.

Answering his own question about whether he could secure support to help with his benefit claim, he writes: 'I have had support before, to get me on these benefits in the first place and to try and help me attend the assessments. I no longer have that support, and I really cannot be bothered to keep trying, or to keep feeling bad for taking up other people's time and resources.'

Although he requests that those reading his letter do not try to persuade him to change his mind, he suggests they contact the DWP 'and let them know why another of their former claimants is ending their life'.

Despite Roy's pleas, a friend alerts the police. He agrees to be taken to the local accident and emergency department, and is admitted to the Campbell Centre. He explains that, despite frequent suicidal thoughts, he has been feeling comfortable with his life in the last few years and has not been actively suicidal. But he then speaks about 'how upset he felt about losing his benefits', and his wish to end his life.

David Marchevsky, the consultant psychiatrist who assesses him, says later that Roy told him he 'did not want to create a fuss or drain resources. We tried to persuade him to accept help with his benefits, but he did not appear very hopeful.' Roy is cooperative, polite and pleasant, smiling and making jokes but 'became tearful when talking about the reasons for being here and about losing his benefits'.

A support worker begins liaising with DWP, passing on a letter from Marchevsky, and within days his ESA is reinstated. When Roy is told, he stops expressing thoughts about dying. He is discharged on 5 October. But within days, DWP sends him another letter. He has been placed back in the work-related activity group and will need to attend regular face-to-face appointments.

On 18 October, he asks the mental health home treatment team to send a supporting letter to DWP, and they suggest he asks his GP. On 12 November, DWP tells him he will need to attend another face-to-face assessment on 3 December. This, DWP admits later, was a letter automatically generated by its IT system.

Roy visits his GP on 15 November, and asks for a letter so he can request a home assessment. The GP agrees to write a letter, but there is nothing in his notes to show any attempt to assess whether Roy is having suicidal thoughts, or if he collected the letter. At some point in the next few days, probably on 18 November, Roy takes his own life in his bedroom, in exactly the way he had promised two months earlier.

The indignities and abuse do not end there. Various agencies, including social services and the housing association, try to contact him. While he was in the Campbell Centre, a social worker had requested an urgent adult social care assessment, attaching a copy of his suicide letter. But Milton Keynes council only allocates a social worker assistant to his case, and not until 26 November. By this time, Roy is already dead.

It is not until 3 December that the assistant social worker makes the first attempt to reach Roy, but only through letters and phone calls, to the wrong number. No visits are made to his flat, and one letter warns that if he fails to make contact by the end of the month, his case will be closed. The case is eventually closed by Milton Keynes council the following month, without a single visit to his flat.

When his ESA stops, so does his rent. Roy's housing association, the Guinness Partnership, fails to check on his welfare for several months, even though he has previously lived in supported accommodation.

In January 2019, DWP stops Roy's ESA, after making two unsuccessful visits to his flat to ask why he had not attended the WCA. The DWP officer notices letters alerting Roy to the visit still in the mailbox. Neighbours have reported the build-up of mail to the housing association. DWP apparently makes no further effort to check on Roy's welfare or contact other agencies, despite his long history of mental distress and suicidal ideation.

In April 2019, the Guinness Partnership issues an eviction notice. The following month, a member of staff visits the flat, but receives no response. She slides a calling card under the door.

Three more months pass. It is not until 21 August that the housing association sends two staff members, a bailiff, a locksmith, and a gas engineer to Roy's flat to evict him. There is no answer when they knock, so the locksmith drills the lock. The flat is clean and tidy. There is a small amount of washing-up, and clothes in the washing machine. There is food in the fridge with 'best before' dates of early December 2018. An open carton of milk in the fridge has a 'use by' date of 22 November 2018. The bailiff finds Roy in his bedroom, in the same position he has been in since taking his life nine months earlier.

* * *

When the inquest takes place late the following year, it provides a detailed inquiry into the events that led to Roy's death, with one exception: no witnesses from DWP or Maximus give evidence.

The coroner is Tom Osborne, who ten years earlier had issued a prevention of future deaths report following the suicide of Stephen Carré. But this time, despite being told about the notes scrawled in red ink across the DWP letters found in Roy's flat, Osborne fails to probe the role of DWP or the work capability assessment in his death. The inquest hears from social services, mental health and housing agencies who describe how DWP's actions contributed to causing Roy's death, but there is no attempt by the coroner to examine those failings.

Osborne concludes that, on the balance of probabilities, Roy took his own life on or about 18 November 2018. He says he will produce a prevention of future deaths report, but will only address it to Milton Keynes City Council, for the failures of its social services department.

Roy's mother, Anabela, tells me afterwards that, although she is 'very grateful' for the coroner's sympathy, fairness and thoroughness, she is 'surprised and disappointed' at the lack of DWP evidence. DWP, she says, repeatedly failed her son. Fuad tells me the notes his son left behind 'tell the story of his struggle with DWP', and he adds: 'DWP policies need to change. Too many lives have been lost.'

A spokesperson for the coroner tells me that 'as an independent judicial office holder' it would be 'inappropriate for him to comment' on why he failed to bring DWP witnesses to give evidence.

* * *

A year later, a few days before Christmas 2021, the *Dispatches* documentary airs on Channel 4.[1] *The Truth about Disability Benefits* features interviews with four of the families I have worked with: Joy Dove and her grand-daughter Emma; Alison and Lee, Errol's son; Imogen Day, and Philippa's mother Jane; and Roy's mother Anabela.

I have been pushing for this documentary to be made for three years, and it is directed, produced, and presented by disabled writer, film-maker and artist Richard Butchins, who has been responsible for a series of critically-acclaimed documentaries exposing DWP and its assessment process, and with whom I've worked on a number of investigative projects. In December 2022, our documentary will win an award at the British Journalism Awards.

Anabela tells Richard that DWP's actions were 'appalling'. 'I believe that what triggered my son to carry on, go ahead with his suicide even though his benefits were reinstated, it was the letters that he kept receiving from DWP reminding [him] that he had to go for the work assessment,' she says. 'There's so many things that can be improved, and it must never happen again, it should never happen again.'

And yet it does. I continue to write about the deaths. Philip Pakree, who had grown increasingly anxious and in fact 'nearly hysterical' as the date of his work capability assessment approached, died on Boxing Day 2020.[2] Sophia Yuferev,[3] whose body was found in her flat in November 2021, months after all her benefits were removed, and who DWP had hounded for years. Christian Wilcox,[4] who had been writing online for several months before his suicide in November 2019 about the impact of the PIP reassessment process on his mental health.

These are some of the deaths I hear about, but the scores of internal process reviews still taking place (54 IPRs into deaths begun in 2019–20, 49 in 2020–21, 47 in 2021–22[5]) show there are many, many others I don't. The department continues its delaying tactics, even branding me 'vexatious' for trying to secure redacted copies of the latest IPRs, and arguing that releasing them would interfere with the development of government policy. When they are finally released, they show how systemic safeguarding flaws across the department continue to be linked to serious harm and deaths.

Several reports between 2018 and 2020 show continuing failings in how DWP staff respond to claimants who disclose ideas of suicide, with one warning of the need for staff to 'show more compassion'. Others completed between September 2020 and November 2022 refer to multiple errors and policy failings across universal credit, ESA, and PIP. The same systemic issues keep reappearing: poor quality assessment reports, the failure to seek evidence from doctors, the refusal to use all available sources of evidence in deciding a claim, poor training …

There are many near misses, too. In October 2022, a disabled man tells me he was left needing hospital treatment three times for suicidal thoughts caused by the actions of jobcentres and universal credit advisers.[6] A legal document describes how the man, from east London, was failed scores of times by DWP staff who refused to communicate with him by phone, rather than through his online universal credit journal, ignored or refused his requests for support, and failed to put markers on his universal credit account to alert colleagues that he was a 'vulnerable claimant'. DWP admits discriminating against him on numerous occasions.

The violence cannot be separated from the department. As Dr China Mills will argue, the harm caused by the actions of DSS – and then DWP – accumulates over the years, and it is attritional. Time, she says, can camouflage this slow, bureaucratic violence, but when you bring the years of evidence together, there it is in the open. She began to see this, and, working with Healing Justice Ldn, which works with marginalised communities in London to address the harm caused by oppression, is determined to show the damage caused by the department.

Working with Rick Burgess, Ellen Clifford, Nick Dilworth, and Dolly Sen, China and I create what she calls the Deaths by Welfare timeline.[7] It brings together government reports, academic research, disabled people's activism, letters to DWP from coroners, media reports, freedom of information responses, and political speeches.

Even without the National Archives documents, which have not yet been added, the timeline shows how years of warning signs were ignored, and demonstrates systemic negligence by DWP, a culture of cover-up and denial, and a refusal to accept that the department has a duty of care to disabled people claiming support through the social security system. It shows how DWP continues to pose a serious risk to the lives of disabled people who pass through its assessment systems. But it also shows how the campaigning and leadership of disabled people and bereaved families has been vital in resisting DWP's violence.

* * *

I speak to Dame Anne McGuire in late June 2023 about her three years as a DWP minister between 2005 and 2008. Her focus had been on furthering disability rights across government as minister for disabled people (she was not responsible for the WCA). Towards the end of our interview, I ask whether her party must accept some of the blame attached to the WCA, which was introduced in 2008 under a Labour government. 'If we did anything that made matters worse for people, in spite of our intention, then I think, you know, we can regret that,' she says. 'I think we did try to change the culture. We tried to introduce a system that was more supportive of people, and I don't think it was particularly easy. You were trying to change something that had been in place for many years. You were trying to [achieve] attitudinal changes within the department.

'Deaths, you know, as a result of something that government does or doesn't do, are awful. And that's a terrible burden for anybody to carry.'

I ask if she thinks the culture at DWP was possibly worse than she thought at the time, and the insurance industry maybe more influential, and that those issues had been there, in the background, unknown to her. 'It probably was. It probably was. Maybe I was touchingly naïve,' she says. She thinks these 'big beasts from the insurance industry' were interested in 'getting a share of the action … They're big businesses. That's what they do. They grow their business, and it's up to politicians to put down the lines over which they will not cross.'

One or two of the families I have met and grown to admire so much over the years occasionally meet each other, usually online, or sometimes at political events or protests. But such contact is rare until the autumn of 2021. For more than a year I have been working with critically acclaimed theatre director Sacha Wares on a ground-breaking digital exhibition which she has designed to recreate the circumstances that led to some of the deaths.

'Museum of Austerity' uses the families' verbal testimony – and 'volumetric capture' techniques that have produced high-quality holograms – to recreate the circumstances that led to the deaths of eight claimants in the decade of austerity from 2010.

My role has been as co-editor and specialist adviser, supporting some of the families I have been working with to tell their stories once again, and record their interviews.* When Sacha and her team are ready to show a work-in-progress version of the exhibition for the first time – at the BFI London Film Festival – the families are invited to London to see it, and to meet each other.

Several of the families meet at a central London hotel as guests of the English Touring Theatre, the National Theatre's Immersive Storytelling Studio, and Sacha's Trial & Error Studio, which have produced the exhibition. They spend hours sharing their experiences.

Errol's son Lee says the exhibition is the first time he has listened to his wife, Alison, being interviewed about his father's death, which includes her description of identifying his body. 'When I heard her speaking and the rawness of it, that really hit me because I didn't know how much she had been suffering,' he says.

Alison adds: 'When you walk in that room, everything just hits you. It's overwhelming, but I don't regret it at all. For that 30 minutes, I didn't feel alone. To be in the room with people who are suffering exactly as you are, you feel normal.'

* * *

Despite the years of research into DWP violence, there was still little to show why lower-ranked civil servants had acted as they had, allowing the hostile environment created by ministers and senior civil servants over three decades to fester and flourish.

In March 2021, research by Dr Jamie Redman and Professor Del Roy Fletcher from Sheffield Hallam University finally shows how that happened.[8] They describe how DWP staff and managers inflicted psychological harm on benefit claimants, engaged in unofficial sanctioning targets, and pushed disabled people into work despite the risks to their health.

---

* With the kind permission of the producers and the families featured, material from these interviews has been used in this book.

The evidence comes from new interviews with ten civil servants who worked for DWP and its contractors between 2010 and 2015. They build on the work of Polish sociologist Zygmunt Bauman, who showed how modern bureaucracies can produce psychosocial factors that enable ordinary people to carry out harmful practices.

They describe how a change in DWP policy under the Conservative-Liberal Democrat coalition pressured staff to refer more claimants to have their benefits sanctioned. Policy changes also saw the performance of jobcentre staff measured by 'off-benefit flows', the number of claimants who stopped receiving an out-of-work benefit, even if they had not secured a job. This led to a huge increase in sanctioning rates between 2010 and 2013 – reaching more than one million sanctions in 2013, about 345 per cent above their 2001–08 average level.

They were told how this 'top-down' pressure on staff acted as a 'moral anaesthetic' which 'made invisible the needs and interests' of the claimants they were sanctioning. Former DWP staff said there was increasing expectation 'from above' to hand out sanctions, which led to the formation of 'local target regimes'.

One jobcentre worker describes how staff would treat claimants with 'disrespect' and use psychological harm as a technique to reduce the number of claimants, 'pushing them until they either just cleared off because they couldn't take the pressure or they got sanctioned'.

But these tactics were not restricted to jobcentres. Those who worked for outsourced Work Programme providers described how managers pressured them to 'push' disabled people into work. One former Work Programme adviser said: '[I had] a lovely guy who I really felt for who had mental health issues and the day after I had to reluctantly mandate him to something – he attempted suicide. I also had another lady who we pushed into work and it made her that ill she had a fit in her new job and was admitted to hospital.'

Another Work Programme adviser said some colleagues seemed to thrive on their ability to inflict harm. Redman and Fletcher said their research sought to explain 'how ordinary people carrying out their daily duties' were able to 'implement cruel and inhumane social security reforms'.

In November 2021, I speak to an autistic man, David Scott, who provides his own example of this cruelty.[9] I listen to a secret recording made by David, in which I can hear comments made by his work coach. During their conversation, David explains that previous treatment he has received from DWP left him suicidal. The conversation appears to be approaching a successful conclusion, as the work coach agrees he will not need to carry out any work-related commitments, other than taking steps to prepare for the start of a PhD in neuroscience the following April.

But when he thanks her, she tells him: 'So I am here to support you whether you like it or you don't, right?' Scott replies that this would be his first experience of such support from DWP. The work coach tells him: 'I'm not here to stick pins in your eyes, unless you want me to. And it will be a Biro, not pins, all right?'

David, who also has long-term health conditions, appears to laugh nervously, but he doesn't otherwise respond. The work coach adds: 'I taught autistic children for a long time, so yeah, it will be a sharp poke.'

David is taking legal action against DWP over the treatment he has received as a disabled claimant of universal credit. In one of his legal letters, he tells DWP's lawyers he is 'routinely treated badly' because he is autistic, and that the key reason he had decided to seek an autism diagnosis was to protect himself from DWP.

I am shown a letter from the Government Legal Department which denies any discrimination but apologises for the work coach's 'inappropriate and misjudged comment'. DWP refuses to comment when I ask if the case illustrates the toxic, hostile, and discriminatory environment frequently faced by disabled people who have to engage with the department.

In March 2022, I am contacted by a DWP whistleblower, who tells me that harsh new policies which are forcing more disabled people to attend weekly face-to-face jobcentre meetings could lead to claimants taking their own lives.

The work coach says she and her colleagues are being 'bullied and harassed' into forcing claimants with significant mental distress into attending work-related meetings. Many have been waiting months for a work capability assessment and will eventually be found not fit for work and placed in universal credit's limited capability for work-related activity group (the equivalent of the old ESA support group). But until that happens, they are being forced to make weekly trips to the jobcentre, purely so work coaches can meet targets for face-to-face appointments. It will not be long before her concerns are realised.

Just weeks later, a disabled woman left traumatised by the daily demands of the universal credit system takes her own life. Days earlier she had been told she would need to attend a face-to-face meeting with a work coach. Rebecca (*not her real name*), a former senior manager for an international publishing company, would shake and cry every time she had to log onto her online universal credit 'journal', which she had to do every weekday to check whether she had received any instructions and avoid a sanction. Although a six-month 'fit note' from her doctor explained she was not fit for work, she was still expected to have regular work coach appointments until Maximus could assess her fitness for work.

DWP had been told of her mental distress, suicidal thoughts and fear of the department and the universal credit system. Her mother, Debra (*not her real name*), told me later that the idea of always having to be under the surveillance of DWP and universal credit left her daughter in despair. She had told her mother: 'They will always want to know where I am going, how much money I have got. They will always be in my life, they will always want to know.'

She was so concerned that she might be sanctioned that she did not turn on the central heating in her flat for the last two months of her life, to try to save money. She wouldn't allow her parents to pay the bill in case DWP saw the payment in her bank account and treated it as income.

Her mother would take food to her daughter's home several times a week, and Rebecca's partner – who did not live with her – was feeding her in the evenings, but the severe anxiety had caused her to lose weight.

The local mental health service provider had persuaded DWP to allow Rebecca's appointment with a work coach on 8 April 2022 to take place by phone, with a support worker with her at home. But the work coach told her: 'We have let you off this time, but you will come to the jobcentre next time.' Just a week later, she took her own life. By the time she died, she weighed less than five stone.

Rebecca was likely to have been declared not fit for work, but she had been waiting for a work capability assessment since completing a questionnaire in January. She was dreading the process. 'The DWP knew my daughter and they knew she was frightened of the DWP,' says Debra. 'Every time you mentioned the jobcentre and DWP, there were tears.' Debra does not want her daughter identified until an inquest takes place, but she has asked the coroner to investigate the role DWP and the universal credit system played in her death.

Debra is clear that it was not universal credit that caused her daughter's depression, but she is certain it was the 'final straw'. A previous experience of claiming universal credit three years ago had left her traumatised. 'She was just petrified of universal credit, of breaking the rules and going to jail. She was just panicking about everything, but universal credit was the thing that was pushing her and pushing her.'

The following year, another case exposes the pressures imposed by the new universal credit system. Kevin Gale was a window-cleaner whose worsening mental health led to him being sectioned. After his discharge in January 2022, he needs financial support from universal credit. But the anxiety caused by his claim instead increases his anxiety and he takes his own life on 4 May. Coroner Kirsty Gomersal writes a prevention of future deaths report to DWP,[10] pointing to the 'number of and length' of the universal credit forms, which 'can be overwhelming for someone with a mental health illness', and which are 'perpetuated if the applicant cannot get help to complete the paperwork', while also highlighting the 'long telephone queues to speak to a DWP advisor'.

After the coroner's office emails me a recording of the inquest, it reveals how senior figures at the mental health trust that had been supporting Kevin warned that the 'debilitating' impact of DWP's actions on people with mental distress was a 'national issue'. They said Gale had repeatedly told mental health professionals about the anxiety his universal credit claim was causing him.

Dr Judith Whiteley, a psychiatrist with the Cumbria, Northumberland, Tyne and Wear NHS Foundation Trust, told the inquest of the impact of DWP's 'inefficiencies', saying: 'It perpetuates their illnesses, their depressions continue, their anxieties continue, and they don't respond to medication as well as they should, the ability to function from day-to-day. Often, they're living on pennies. They can't afford to feed themselves properly.'

* * *

I am contacted in the summer of 2022 by Stephen Carré's daughter Jennifer – Jen. She has been speaking with her aunt, Sarah, after finding her on Facebook, and wants to discover more about what happened to her father. She is now 21, and only found out when she was 18 that he had taken his own life. She has been researching not only my stories on Stephen's death, but those on other deaths linked to DWP. She has a lot of questions, not least how her dad could have been betrayed so badly by the department.

I tell her as much as I can, and over the following months she emails occasionally. She knows little about her dad, as she was so young when he died, and he had not been able to visit in the last few years of his life. She has mostly got to know Stephen 'through the memories of others'.

She knows he carried out 'extensive research' before she was born. 'He would research the best cot and the best food and the best everything in preparation,' she says. 'He made sure to work hard in and out of work to provide for us, and it meant that I had everything I would have ever needed when I was very young.' She also shares with me the few memories of her own. 'I remember him occasionally letting me try his beer and pull his glasses off his head to try them on. He never got mad at me. Instead, he found it hilarious.'

Later, she knew how different she was from other children. 'I remember other kids laughing at me for only having one parent, and thinking it was my fault,' she tells me. 'I am lucky to have a very supportive mum that helped me through this.'

She finds out about his suicide just as she is about to start university, almost ten years after he died. She begins to connect with relatives on Stephen's side of the family. At first, she is angry. At her relatives, at DWP, and because she could not understand why this happened.

'It was surreal hearing from relatives that I had never really spoken to before,' she says. She is surprised to hear they had been thinking about her and her brother, and had been keeping tabs on them through Facebook. Reconnecting with Stephen's relatives has led to her being sent many pictures of her dad. 'It's strange that I don't recognise him, or anyone in the pictures,' she tells me.

She is angry at the 'multiple inexcusable errors' that led to his suicide, at the lack of protection for disabled people, and the benefit scrounger rhetoric spouted by politicians like Iain Duncan Smith. She is upset, also, when she learns how Stephen's father, Peter, felt pushed to bring his son's ashes to the posthumous ESA appeal hearing, and when she learns that DWP eventually found her dad not fit for work, but only after he had killed himself.

'It's hard to imagine what life could have been like if they had reached this conclusion originally,' she says. 'Would myself and my brother have had Stephen in our lives? Would our lives be different?'

She tells me that seeing all the information about the deaths that has been collected over the years, and how other families have been impacted, makes her feel almost helpless. 'It's shocking to think that they have repeatedly made the same mistake and cost other people their lives, and that little to no changes have been made after all of this,' she says.

'I cannot begin to imagine all of the other families and friends going through the same thing as us. The volume of anger and grief from something so avoidable is astounding, and yet there is no change. It makes you think about how long this will go on for, and how many other lives will be lost.'

Epilogue

When I speak to Mansel Aylward – now Professor Sir Mansel Aylward – in March 2023, he has recently returned from an international lecture tour. It is the first time we have spoken since a brief conversation at a conference in 2012. Now 80 years old, he is intent on securing his legacy. He is proud of his leading role in devising the all work test. It was, he says, his claim to fame. We speak for more than two-and-a-half hours.

This conversation is a missing piece in the DWP puzzle. His memory is sharp. He is complimentary about those he worked with in the department, including Peter Lilley. And when I ask him about deaths linked to the all work test, he thinks there were just four or five, but says he does not remember any suicides, even those of Dermot Comiskey and Kevin Shields from early 1997.

When I tell him that hundreds of deaths were later linked to the WCA, he nearly shouts down the phone. 'Hundreds of deaths!?' he cries. 'I didn't know that.' He says these figures worry him. He insists that nothing like this happened with the all work test. 'I don't know what's happened,' he says. His first suggestion is that the assessment is being 'applied too rigorously' and those who carry out the assessments are maybe not being monitored. 'The figures you quote to me are, you know, I just don't understand, something's gone wrong. It didn't happen [before]. Why is it happening now?'

He is also astonished when I tell him DWP now allows healthcare professionals such as nurses and paramedics to carry out the assessments. 'I made it quite clear that they had to be a medically qualified person: doctors, physicians and surgeons,' he says.

'You've educated me to something,' he says. 'I have to do some background reading, obviously, but I don't want something that I was associated with in developing being a cause of so much stress that people commit suicide. I abhor that, you know? It's terrible.'

He promises to contact the DWP civil servant who is now in his former role of chief medical officer.

> I would like to know what the qualifications are of people who are doing an assessment. I want to know what training they had beforehand. I want to know how much they're monitored thereafter, and I'd like to know if he would explain to me why there are so many deaths. Because he must know, mustn't he? Well, we want to look into it so you can, you know, put that element into your book as well.

He tells me he knows the assessment system deteriorated after he left, but, he says, 'I'm not going to go into that.' He makes a further comment about this later in our interview but asks me not to include it. Clearly something happened in the 2000s, around the time he left DWP, but he won't say what it was.

When I ask if he believes disability analysists can assess disabled people accurately for their eligibility for benefits, he says:

> I can't talk for the recent years, but when I was there, yes, absolutely yes. We checked up on them, we looked at the results of their decisions, and I was satisfied that that was OK. I never had a problem with things like that because… I met with all the doctors that were working, and they had regular updates. They had regular revision sessions when I was there. And I don't know what happened subsequently… if they weren't doing that, I would've been upset.

We agreed to speak again once he had researched some of my concerns.

It is a fascinating conversation, but it leaves important questions unanswered. What were his disagreements with DWP – possibly with ministers – in the 2000s? And what would he discover if he talked to his successor at DWP? He sounded genuinely shocked and concerned when I told him of the hundreds of suicides linked to the WCA, although I found it odd that someone who lectured around the world on his work, and was still working two days a week at Cardiff University, had not been aware of the deaths linked to the WCA.

He says he will carry out some research before talking to me again. He asks me to send him some background information. However, soon after our conversation, he becomes seriously unwell and needs an emergency operation for pancreatic cancer. When I speak to his wife in July 2023, she tells me he probably has just months or even weeks to live, but that he still wants to 'set the record straight'. She asks me to email across some follow-up questions. He had not responded by the time this book went to press.

* * *

In March 2023, ministers announce plans to scrap the work capability assessment.[1] Although this secures widespread support in the mainstream media, that approval is not shared by disabled people who know how the system works.

The proposal is that, instead of the WCA deciding eligibility for out-of-work disability benefits, an extra 'health element' will be awarded to anyone receiving both universal credit and personal independence payment. But, as activists point out, the PIP assessment is just as troubling a process as the WCA.

But there is more to it than that. The proposals – which it is hoped will only be implemented if the Conservatives win the next election – mean it would be up to jobcentre work coaches to decide if a disabled person can carry out work-related activity such as attending regular job-focused interviews or taking part in a training course. When Peter Lilley introduced the all work test in 1995, these decisions were – essentially – taken by doctors, although they were signed off by DWP civil servants. In 2008, with the introduction of the WCA, it was decided that paramedics, physiotherapists, and nurses could also carry out the assessments and provide the necessary advice to DWP. But DWP is now arguing that work coaches with no healthcare training at all will be able to decide if a disabled person is able to take part in work-related activity. It is another dangerous backwards step, particularly in the light of evidence emerging in late 2023 of the significant workload pressures being imposed on DWP staff. The Public and Commercial Services Union presents a dossier of evidence[2] from its members to DWP which it says shows the department is in a 'state of crisis' and faces a 'near collapse' of its benefits systems. The union accuses DWP of 'deliberate neglect', after its members said they believed benefit claimants in vulnerable situations were 'falling through the gaps' in the system. One manager says staff are facing 'completely overwhelming' workloads.

The department takes another dangerous step, with plans to further tighten the work capability assessment in the lead-up to its eventual abolition. The final plans, following a much-criticised consultation, include tightening the 'substantial risk' safety net so it only applies in 'exceptional circumstances', protecting those with 'the most severe mental or physical health conditions'.[3]

Chancellor Jeremy Hunt later says it is 'wrong economically and wrong morally' to provide support for so many disabled people without forcing them to look for work. The changes will cut DWP spending by an estimated £1.265 billion a year by 2028–29 and will mean 371,000 disabled people losing up to £390 a month and becoming subject to strict conditions and sanctions. The WCA reforms will increase employment by just 10,000 by 2028–29, according to the Office for Budget Responsibility.[4]

And what of Unum? Since its incessant – and effective – lobbying of DWP from the 1990s to the 2010s, it has retreated into the shadows around disability benefit reform. I find a reference in Hansard from 2018, when the SNP's Carol Monaghan spoke in a Commons debate[5] of Unum's links to the notorious PACE trial. The flawed trial was partly funded by DWP and assumed that ME (myalgic encephalomyelitis) was psychological and that those with the condition 'could recover if they chose so to do', Monaghan told fellow MPs.

'When we consider the relationship between key PACE investigators and major health insurance companies such as Unum,' Monaghan said, 'the trial takes on a far more sinister slant.' She said that people with ME had reported that their health insurance company would pay out only if they undertook a programme of graded exercise therapy, where physical activity is gradually increased over time, no matter how the patient is responding.

It is a reminder that the 'illness behaviours' theory and the biopsychosocial model promoted by Mansel Aylward were still being used by the insurance industry to deny valid claims but were also still embedded in DWP culture. As Monaghan told MPs: 'One wonders why the DWP would fund such a trial, unless it was seen as a way of removing people from long-term benefits and reducing the welfare bill.'

Since this debate, there has not been a single mention of Unum reported by Hansard. Perhaps it feels its work has been done.

* * *

In *The Violence of Austerity*,[6] Vickie Cooper and David Whyte write of how institutional violence differs from street robberies and muggings in dark alleys. 'The violence of austerity is delivered by smartly dressed people sitting behind desks,' they write. And who are those we should blame, they ask? The politicians, the civil servants, the government departments, and the local authorities. 'And in front of them stand the armies of private officials in companies like G4S and ATOS and public officials in benefit offices and housing trusts.'

It's crucial to remember that the violence described in *The Department* did not stand alone in the austerity years. As *The Violence of Austerity* shows, the impact was spread across society: the asylum system, children and young people's services, the environment, health and safety, housing evictions, the criminal justice system, street homelessness…

But I believe that the violence perpetrated by the department, both under its DSS and DWP brandings, was different. It was the result of a particular combination of time, hostility, bureaucratic arrogance and opacity, greed and political opportunism.

Disabled researcher and writer Sue Jones would say in early 2023[7] that it had now 'become the norm for the DWP to inflict psychological injury on the citizens it is meant to support'. Discussing the death of Philippa Day, she said the social security system was 'a hostile environment, it promotes a culture of systemic disbelief towards the very people it is supposed to support'. Jones had written six years earlier[8] of how our former liberal democracy had been transformed into an authoritarian state 'that values production, competition and profit above all else'.

Within months of the announcement of the scrapping of the WCA, there is another demonstration of DWP's willingness, and even eagerness, to inflict psychological harm on its claimants. Stories begin to appear in the national media. They seem to be part of a re-emerging DWP strategy of undermining public sympathy for the social security system, now the pandemic and the threat of destitution is no longer at the front of the average citizen's mind. Articles begin to emerge in the media, just as they did in January 1990 with the '£4bn row over "lead swinging"' and the 'Scandal of sick notes'. And just as they did in 2010 when *The Sun* was telling its readers – through Iain Duncan Smith – that they were 'right to be angry' when they saw neighbours who did not work.

Jeremy Vine's Channel 5 television show is one of the first to support the DWP strategy,[9] publishing a social media post – later deleted – that asks if it is wrong for 'taxpayers' to pay 'indefinitely' for the benefits of those 'deemed too sick to work'.

The Telegraph is again among the culprits,[10] telling its readers that 'Millions are claiming benefits without ever having to look for work' and producing an automatic calculator that allows readers to discover 'just how much of our hard-won salaries are spent on the benefits of those who do not work' (the article is softened slightly after an outcry). Natasha Hirst, the disabled president of the National Union of Journalists, says the recent reporting 'has reinforced a damaging narrative that blames and punishes disabled people for situations that are not of their making'.

Leading the way is the latest Conservative minister for disabled people, Tom Pursglove, who posts a hostile and 'dangerous' post on social media[11] that warns fraudulent benefit claimants that DWP will 'track you down' and 'bring you to justice'. The video – posted by DWP on Twitter and by Pursglove on his Facebook page – is a clumsy parody of a speech in the violent Liam Neeson thriller *Taken*, in which Neeson's character promises: 'I will look for you, I will find you, and I will kill you.' In the DWP video, Pursglove says to camera: 'We will track you down. We will find you. And we will bring you to justice.'

As disabled activist and consultant clinical psychologist Dr Jay Watts says:

> The DWP video not only plays on fears of persecution and being accused of wrongdoing, which claimants tell us in clinic provokes terror, despair, and anxiety – quite understandably, unfortunately, given the cruelty of our current welfare system – but also ramps up the messaging with highly evocative and persecutory language almost perfectly designed to trigger fear responses in the body. When I say that this policy will get inside people's heads in terms of intrusive thoughts and persecutory auditory hallucinations, I mean it quite literally.

In July 2023, thanks particularly to years of pressure from Labour's Debbie Abrahams, the Commons work and pensions committee announces an inquiry into how DWP supports 'vulnerable claimants' and its approach to safeguarding. Should it have a statutory safeguarding duty? Is DWP transparent enough about deaths linked to its actions? And how successful is the internal process review in investigating deaths, and how well does the department implement the recommendations from these secret reviews?

It is not the independent, statutory, public inquiry that many want to see, but it is at least the first serious public investigation into safeguarding at the department since reports of deaths first began emerging in the early 2010s. Its conclusions were due to be published as this book went to press. One thing is clear, though: it will not provide justice for those who have died.

* * *

The department continues to delay and block information about its failings. It refuses to release a report on 'the impact of errors on vulnerable customers', and a document that would show how its plans to scrap the WCA would impact disabled people.

In July, China Mills and I publish a well-received article (China is very much the lead author) that shows how DWP has 'weaponised' time as a strategy to avoid being held accountable for benefit-related deaths.[12] It shows how the department's use of delaying tactics helped deny justice to the relatives of those who died, and draws heavily on the Deaths by Welfare timeline, and my decade-long freedom of information battle with the department.

As Rick Burgess says in a Deaths by Welfare event in January 2023, this is 'a history that the state would prefer that no-one wrote down, that no-one paid attention to, because it is state-sanctioned harm'. As a survivor of the assessment system, he believes that for victims, survivors, and other disabled people to feel that things have changed, the department must be abolished. He also believes there should be a truth and reconciliation process, while some individuals 'absolutely should end up behind bars'. This is, after all, large-scale state violence. 'I think it needs to be said that that level of harm has been reached, that level of trauma has been reached,' he says.

How many people died as a direct result of this DWP slow violence? We will never know. From that first memo early in 1989 that spoke of 'the need to tackle the rising expenditure on these benefits', fairness and justice were slowly, week by week, year by year, replaced with indifference and cruelty. Evidence was replaced by guesswork and prejudice. It led to distress and poverty, to sanctions and starvation, to psychological torture and suicide.

Can we allow those responsible for this breakdown of fairness and justice to escape without accountability?

As Rick Burgess suggests, we need truth and reconciliation. If there is no such process, the pain, the misery, the horror, will remain a thick mass hanging permanently above our machinery of government, our social security system, and its guardian: the Department for Work and Pensions.

But as he says, we need more than that. In the name of the countless hundreds, and almost certainly thousands, who have lost their lives, there must also now – after decades of dehumanising bureaucratic neglect, cruelty and violence – be justice.

Acknowledgements

It is not false modesty to say that this book would not have been possible without the courage and dedication of countless disabled people and allies. I can't name them all but thank you to every one of them who has helped with my research at Disability News Service (DNS). I must also thank all those who have supported DNS and kept it afloat for the last 15 years, both my wonderful subscribers and others who have contributed financially and with their kind words and actions.

I only began my own serious investigations into DWP a couple of years after disabled people's grassroots groups had begun to raise their concerns about the violent impact of government austerity. It was their research that inspired me to do more to examine what was really happening within the Department for Work and Pensions, and, later, what had happened in the previous two decades.

The grassroots groups and disabled people's organisations that have played vital roles in exposing this wrongdoing include (in alphabetical order) Black Triangle, Chronic Illness Inclusion, Disability Rights UK, Disabled People Against Cuts (DPAC), Inclusion London, the Mental Health Resistance Network, Pat's Petition, Recovery in the Bin, Spartacus, the War on Welfare (WOW) campaign, and WinVisible. I will resist naming too many individuals as I know they value solidarity rather than individual acclaim, but it would be wrong not to mention Linda Burnip and the late Debbie Jolly, both co-founders of DPAC.

Thanks also to two law firms that have done so much to hold DWP to account in the courts: Leigh Day (particularly Merry Varney) and Public Law Project; to Alex Wade, from Reviewed & Cleared, for some useful informal guidance; to data protection expert Jon Baines, from Mishcon de Reya, and barrister Elizabeth Kelsey, for their expert pro bono work in prising information from DWP; and to staff at the National Archives, and Jayne Hale at Tredegar Library, for their help.

There are some other individuals I must mention, for their invaluable help and support at various points during this grim journey, including Ellen Clifford, without whom this book would probably not have been published, Dr Jay Watts, John McArdle, Annie Howard and John Slater, Mary Wilkinson, Owen Stevens, Mo Stewart, Professor Sally McManus, now at the Violence and Society Centre, and Rick Burgess; also Kate Ginn and Annie Brown (both fine journalists and even finer friends) for their perceptive and valuable comments on an early draft of this book. And the late, and much-missed, Nick Dilworth.

There are some people I cannot name, because they have always wished to remain anonymous, including several DWP whistleblowers, and I thank them for everything they have done to expose the violence I describe in these pages. The same applies, of course, to anyone I have forgotten to mention. I hope you'll forgive me.

At a relatively late stage in my investigations, three major projects that I worked on propelled me to take the decision to write *The Department*, and provided crucial research material. My thanks to Channel 4's *Dispatches*, Hardcash Productions, and particularly Richard Butchins, whose investigations, talent, and drive helped expose DWP's actions at various key points over the last decade. Also to the amazing Sacha Wares, who asked me to work on her 'Museum of Austerity' mixed reality installation, and provided an opportunity to work with the National Theatre and the English Touring Theatre on a powerful and ground-breaking project. And finally to Dr China Mills, and Healing Justice Ldn, with whom I worked on the *Deaths by Welfare Project*, which now provides a vital, evidenced timeline of DWP harm. China has been a wonderful, supportive friend and colleague on this and other projects.

Thank you so much to Pluto Press for taking a chance on *The Department*, and particularly to my fantastic editor Neda Tehrani, whose skilful and sensitive handling of the manuscript, and her belief in the importance of this story, has made the journey from manuscript to publication so much easier than I expected. Also to

Robert Webb, Elaine Ross, Dave Stanford, and Melanie Patrick in the production department.

And, of course, I must mention the relatives of those who died, who have all generously given their time over many years and trusted me with the stories of their loved ones, and without whom this book could not have been written. With grateful thanks to the families of Stephen Carré, David Clapson, Mark Wood, David Barr, Faiza Ahmed, Michael O'Sullivan, Jodey Whiting, James Oliver, Philippa Day, Errol Graham, and Roy Curtis/Ayman Habayeb, and particularly to Peter Carré, Sarah Carré, Gill Thompson, Jill Gant, David Barr, Mo Ahmed, Anne-Marie O'Sullivan, Joy Dove, Dave Smith, Imogen Day, Alison Burton, and Anabela Sousa. And to all the other friends and relatives of other victims and survivors whose contributions have played such a vital part in exposing DWP.

Finally, I hope all those who have suffered and survived through DWP's actions, and whose stories have never been reported, know that their voices are also part of this book, at least in spirit. I hope its publication offers hope that an end to their ordeal is somewhere this side of the horizon.

Notes

Websites last accessed 29 February 2024.

CHAPTER 1

1. John Moore, confidential draft letter (Department of Social Security (DSS)/National Archives, 1989).
2. Memo (DSS/National Archives, 1992).
3. Social Surveys (Gallup Poll) Ltd, *Long-term Medical Certification* (DSS/National Archives, 1989).
4. Cuttings collected by DSS (DSS/National Archives, 1990).
5. Public Accounts Committee, *22nd Report, 1989–90: Invalidity Benefit* (House of Commons, 1990).
6. *Tribunal Statistics Quarterly: April to June 2022* (Ministry of Justice, 2022).
7. Letter (HM Treasury/National Archives, 7 March 1991).

CHAPTER 2

1. Memo (DSS/National Archives, 15 June 1992).
2. Memo (DSS/National Archives, May 1992).
3. Memo (DSS/National Archives, 15 June 1992).
4. Memo (DSS/National Archives, 4 June 1992).
5. Memo (DSS/National Archives, 12 June 1992).

CHAPTER 3

1. Memo (DSS/National Archives, 22 July 1992).
2. Memo (DSS/National Archives, 14 August 1992).
3. Memo (DSS/National Archives, October 1992).
4. Peter Lilley, speech to Conservative Party conference (October 1992): www.youtube.com/watch?v=FOx8q3eGq3g
5. Memo (DSS/National Archives, November 1992).
6. Peter Lilley (Hansard, 12 November 1992).
7. Memo (DSS/National Archives, 29 April 1993).
8. John Major (Hansard, 15 June 1993).

9. 'IVB Attacks Creating a "Climate of Fear"' (*Disability Now*, November 1993).
10. Peter Lilley, 'Benefits and Costs: Securing the Future of Social Security', in *Policy Makers on Policy: The Mais Lectures*, ed. Forrest Capie and Geoffrey E. Wood (Routledge, July 1993).

CHAPTER 4

1. Peter Lilley (Hansard, 24 January 1994).
2. Nick Wikeley, The Social Security (Incapacity for Work) Act 1994 (*The Modern Law Review*, 1995).
3. Jenny Morris, 'Beveridge Would Be Saying "It's the Economy, Stupid"' (November 2012): https://jennymorrisnet.blogspot.com/2012/11/beveridge-would-be-saying-its-economy.html
4. Memo (DSS/National Archives, 21 November 1994).
5. Memo (DSS/National Archives, 15 September 1994).
6. Press release (DSS/National Archives, 28 September 1994).
7. *The Guardian* (DSS/National Archives, September 1994).
8. Memo (DSS/National Archives, 21 November 1994).

CHAPTER 5

1. Confidential cabinet minutes (Cabinet Office/National Archives, 6 April 1995).
2. Memo (DSS/National Archives, March 1995).
3. Dave Gibbs, 'Incapacity Benefit: A Contradiction That Can't Last' (*Disability Now*, April 1995).
4. 'Lilley Wheelchair "Slur"' (*Disability Now*, June 1995).
5. Paul Foot, 'Doctor on Call' (*Private Eye*, 16 June 1995).
6. Memo (DSS/National Archives, 11 August 1995).
7. Memo (HM Treasury, July 1995).
8. Mansel Aylward and John LoCascio, 'Problems in the Assessment of Psychosomatic Conditions in Social Security Benefits and Related Commercial Schemes' (*Journal of Psychosomatic Research*, August 1995).
9. *The Medical Assessment of Incapacity and Disability Benefits* (National Audit Office, 9 March 2001).
10. Richard Brooks, *Plundering the Public Sector*, by David Craig with Richard Brooks (Constable, 2006).
11. Alan Howarth, *Benefits Agency Medical Service*, early day motion 701 (UK Parliament website, March 1997).
12. Ellen Clifford, *The War on Disabled People* (Zed Books, 2020).

13. Alistair Burt, memo (DSS/National Archives, 14 January 1996).
14. Memo (DSS/National Archives, 13 March 1996).
15. Steve Griffiths, 'Dark Times for Those That Cannot Work' (*Compass*, October 2010).
16. Memo (DSS/National Archives, March 1996).
17. Tom O'Grady, *The Transformation of British Welfare Policy* (Oxford University Press, June 2022).
18. *The System* (BBC2, 1996).
19. 'Incapacity Test Gives Unlucky Break' (*Disability Now*, October 1996).

CHAPTER 6

1. Gordon Caldecott, 'Worried to Death' (*Gwent Gazette*, 14 November 1996).
2. Llew Smith (Hansard, 3 December 1996).
3. Memo (DSS/National Archives, 2 December 1996).
4. Alistair Burt, letter to Llew Smith (DSS/National Archives, 9 December 1996).
5. Alistair Burt, letter to Mansel Aylward (DSS/National Archives, 18 December 1996).
6. Memo (DSS/National Archives, January 1997).
7. Memo (DSS/National Archives, December 1996).
8. Alistair Burt, letter to Frank Field (DSS/National Archives, 11 February 1997).
9. 'An Unfit Test' (National Association of Citizens Advice Bureaux, 3 March 1997).
10. Memo (DSS/National Archives, 28 February 1997).
11. Memo (DSS/National Archives, 12 March 1997).
12. Memo (DSS/National Archives, 24 March 1997).
13. Arthur Delaney, 'Cutting Social Security Disability Benefits Can Backfire Horribly' (*Huffington Post*, 15 January 2020): www.huffingtonpost.co.uk/entry/trump-disability-benefits_n_5e1e3301c5b650c621e71bbc
14. Opinion, 'Work or Die' (*New York Times*, 23 May 1983): www.nytimes.com/1983/05/23/opinion/work-or-die.html
15. 'Labour Turns Big Brother' (*Disability Now*, July 1997).
16. *Social Security – Fourth Report* (Social Security Committee, 13 May 1998).

CHAPTER 7

1. Tom O'Grady, *The Transformation of British Welfare Policy* (Oxford University Press, June 2022).

2. Roger Berry MP, *Benefits Agency Medical Service*, early day motion 65 (House of Commons, 3 June 1997): https://edm.parliament.uk/early-day-motion/16376
3. Confidential cabinet minutes (Cabinet Office/National Archives, 18 December 1997).
4. Harriet Harman (Hansard, 15 December 1997): https://publications.parliament.uk/pa/cm199798/cmhansrd/vo971215/debtext/71215-01.htm#71215-01_spnew9
5. Memo (DSS/National Archives, 1 December 1997).
6. Memo (DSS/National Archives, undated but probably early 1998).
7. Andrew Rawnsley, *Servants of the People* (Penguin Books, 2001).
8. *The Medical Assessment of Incapacity and Disability Benefits* (National Audit Office, 9 March 2001).
9. *New Ambitions for Our Country – A New Contract for Welfare* (government green paper, March 1998).
10. *Social Security – Fourth Report* (Social Security Committee, 13 May 1998).
11. Bob Jessop, 'From Thatcherism to New Labour: Neo-liberalism, Workfarism, and Labour Market Regulation' (Department of Sociology, Lancaster University): www.lancaster.ac.uk/fass/resources/sociology-online-papers/papers/jessop-from-thatcherism-to-new-labour.pdf
12. Libby Brooks, 'In the Workfare State, Poverty Is Always an Individual Failing' (*Guardian*, 11 June 2009).
13. O'Grady, *The Transformation of British Welfare Policy.*
14. Memo (DSS/National Archives, 9 April 1998).
15. Memo (DSS/National Archives, 2 April 1998).
16. Roger Berry (Hansard, 20 May 1999): https://hansard.parliament.uk/commons/1999-05-20/debates/935fd975-15e0-4cd0-9b50-0feefc82bd90/OrdersOfTheDay

CHAPTER 8

1. Mike Wood (Hansard, 16 March 2000): https://hansard.parliament.uk/commons/2000-03-16/debates/6c1d59d2-f269-4ec7-9332-cc8b138c08f3/MentallyIllPeople
2. Memos, letters and statements (DSS/National Archives, 11 August 1999–15 March 2000).
3. *Debate on Permanent Health Insurance* (Hansard, 21 December 1999): https://hansard.parliament.uk/commons/1999-12-21/debates/a7ad345b-dd4a-480d-90b6-2dc21f41f3d1/PermanentHealthInsurance

4. *The Medical Assessment of Incapacity and Disability Benefits* (National Audit Office, 9 March 2001).
5. Alan Hedges and Wendy Sykes, 'Moving between Sickness and Work' (DWP, 2001).
6. Peter Halligan, Christopher Bass and David Oakley (eds), *Malingering and Illness Deception* (Oxford University Press, 2003).
7. Mansel Aylward, 'Origins, Practice, and Limitations of Disability Assessment Medicine', in *Malingering and Illness Deception*, ed. Peter Halligan, Christopher Bass and David Oakley (Oxford University Press, 2003).
8. Gordon Waddell and Mansel Aylward, *Models of Sickness and Disability* (Royal Society of Medicine, 2010).
9. Michael Jones, 'Law, Lies, and Videotape: Malingering as a Legal Phenomenon', in *Malingering and Illness Deception*, ed. Peter Halligan, Christopher Bass and David Oakley (Oxford University Press, 2003).
10. Mansel Aylward and John LoCascio, 'Problems in the Assessment of Psychosomatic Conditions in Social Security Benefits and Related Commercial Schemes' (*Journal of Psychosomatic Research*, August 1995).
11. Jolyon Jenkins, 'Fit for Work' (BBC Radio 4, June 2023).
12. John LoCascio, 'Malingering, Insurance Medicine, and the Medicalization of Fraud', in *Malingering and Illness Deception*, ed. Peter Halligan, Christopher Bass and David Oakley (Oxford University Press, 2003).
13. 'Unum Provident – Story behind the Claims' (Pillsbury & Coleman): www.pillsburycoleman.com/successes/unum-provident-story-behind-the-claims/
14. David Kohn, 'Did Insurer Cheat Disabled Clients?' (CBS News, 14 November 2002).
15. John H. Langbein, 'Trust Law as Regulatory Law: The Unum/Provident Scandal and Judicial Review of Benefit Denials under ERISA' (*Northwestern University Law Review*, 2007).
16. Victoria Colliver, 'State Fines Big Insurer $8 Million' (SFGATE, 3 October 2005): www.sfgate.com/news/article/state-fines-big-insurer-8-million-2566677.php
17. Joanne Hindle, Memorandum Submitted by UnumProvident (Work and Pensions Committee, 13 December 2002): https://publications.parliament.uk/pa/cm200203/cmselect/cmworpen/401/3021203.htm
18. Tom O'Grady, *The Transformation of British Welfare Policy* (Oxford University Press, June 2022).
19. Press release (Cardiff University, May 2004).
20. Memo (DSS/National Archives, undated but likely late 1996).

21. UnumProvident Centre for Psychosocial and Disability Research, newsletter (Cardiff University, 2005): https://issuu.com/maxhead/docs/unum_cardiff_newsletter_issue_1
22. 'Group Income Protection: Evolving the Way We Look at Claims' (UnumProvident, 2005).
23. Gordon Waddell and Mansel Aylward, 'The Scientific and Conceptual Basis of Incapacity Benefits' (DWP, October 2005).
24. Jonathan Rutherford, *New Labour, the Market State, and the End of Welfare* (Soundings, 2007).

CHAPTER 9

1. Jolyon Jenkins, 'Fit for Work' (BBC Radio 4, June 2023).
2. 'Employment of Disabled People 2022' (DWP, 26 January 2023).
3. 'A New Deal for Welfare' (DWP, January 2006).
4. 'What the Doctor Ordered?' (Citizens Advice Bureau, February 2006): https://www.citizensadvice.org.uk/Global/Migrated_Documents/corporate/what-the-doctor-ordered---pdf.pdf
5. Gordon Waddell and Kim Burton, 'Is Work Good for Your Health and Well-being?' (DWP, 2006).
6. Alison Ravetz, 'An Independent Assessment of the Arguments for Proposed Incapacity Benefit Reform (University of Leeds, March 2006): https://disability-studies.leeds.ac.uk/wp-content/uploads/sites/40/library/ravetz-Green-Paper-IB-critique.pdf
7. David Freud, 'Reducing Dependency, Increasing Opportunity' (DWP, March 2007).
8. Welfare Reform Act 2007: www.legislation.gov.uk/ukpga/2007/5/contents
9. Press release (DWP, 19 November 2007): www.wired-gov.net/wg/wg-news-1.nsf/0/73933DF6ABAF730F802573980039FD60?OpenDocument
10. 'Incapacity Benefit Set for Axe' (*Daily Mirror*, 5 November 2007): www.mirror.co.uk/news/uk-news/incapacity-benefit-set-for-axe-518511
11. Patrick Wintour, 'Tiredness among 480 Reasons People Give for Being Unable to Work' (*Guardian*, 19 November 2007): www.theguardian.com/money/2007/nov/19/workandcareers
12. Rachel Sylvester and Alice Thomson, 'Welfare Is a Mess, Says Adviser David Freud' (*Telegraph*, 2 February 2008): www.telegraph.co.uk/news/politics/1577313/Welfare-is-a-mess-says-adviser-David-Freud.html
13. Press release, 'Purnell: New Sanctions Regime for Those Who Try and Play the System' (DWP, 20 February 2008).

14. Helen Hunt, 'Get-Tough Tests Face the Sick on Benefit' (*Liverpool Echo*, 9 April 2008): www.liverpoolecho.co.uk/news/liverpool-news/get-tough-tests-face-sick-benefit-3488200
15. Editorial, 'The Benefits of Welfare Reform Outweigh the Risks' (*Guardian*, 23 November 2008): www.theguardian.com/commentisfree/2008/nov/23/welfare-benefits-economy
16. John Pring, 'Concerns over Tory Incapacity Benefit Plans' (Disability News Service, 30 October 2009): www.disabilitynewsservice.com/concerns-over-tory-incapacity-benefit-plans/
17. Gabriel Milland, '75% on Sick Benefits Are Faking' (*Daily Express*, 14 October 2009): www.express.co.uk/news/uk/133880/75-on-sick-benefits-are-faking
18. John Pring, 'Concerns over First Government Work Test Figures' (Disability News Service, 30 October 2009): www.disabilitynewsservice.com/concerns-over-first-government-work-test-figures/

CHAPTER 10

1. John Pring, 'Figures Show Thousands Missing out on Employment Support' (Disability News Service, 2 January 2010): www.disabilitynewsservice.com/figures-show-thousands-missing-out-on-employment-support/
2. Tom O'Grady, *The Transformation of British Welfare Policy* (Oxford University Press, June 2022).
3. *Work Capability Assessment Internal Review* (DWP, March 2010): https://webarchive.nationalarchives.gov.uk/ukgwa/20130128102031/www.dwp.gov.uk/docs/work-capability-assessment-review.pdf
4. 'Even Harsher New ESA Medical Approved' (Benefits and Work, 13 April 2010): www.benefitsandwork.co.uk/news/even-harsher-new-esa-medical-approved
5. *Building Bridges to Work* (DWP, March 2010): https://assets.publishing.service.gov.uk/government/uploads/system/uploads/attachment_data/file/238471/7817.pdf
6. *Not Working* (Citizens Advice, 23 March 2010).
7. Malcolm Harrington, *Work Capability Assessment Independent Review – Year 1* (DWP, 23 November 2010): www.gov.uk/government/publications/work-capability-assessment-independent-review-year-1
8. *A Future Fair for All* (Labour Party, April 2010).
9. Yvette Cooper, press release (Labour Party, 28 June 2010).
10. John Pring, '"Terrified" Survivors Burn Osborne Effigy in Cuts Protest' (Disability News Service, 31 October 2010): www.disabilitynewsservice.com/terrified-survivors-burn-osborne-effigy-in-cuts-protest/

11. Tom Newton Dunn, 'Shirkers Paradise: IDS on Benefits Britain' (*Sun*, 1 December 2010).
12. 'DWP Panic and Cover-up after Claimant Death Publicity' (Benefits and Work, 13 September 2016): www.benefitsandwork.co.uk/news/dwp-panic-and-cover-up-after-claimant-death-publicity-wca-medics-warned-we-cannot-defend-you

CHAPTER 11

1. 'Response to Call for Evidence' (Mental Health Resistance Network, 16 September 2011).
2. 'Labour's Hypocrisy on "Shirkers vs Workers"' (*Financial Times*, 8 January 2013): www.ft.com/content/584c3ba9-45d0-33c0-b65e-74368c500d6b
3. Emma Briant, Nick Watson and Greg Philo, 'Bad News for Disabled People' (Inclusion London, October 2011): www.inclusionlondon.org.uk/campaigns-and-policy/facts-and-information/equality-and-human-rights/bad-news-for-disabled-people-2
4. Debbie Jolly, 'A Tale of Two Models' (Disabled People Against Cuts, 8 April 2012): https://dpac.uk.net/2012/04/a-tale-of-two-models-disabled-people-vs-unum-atos-government-and-disability-charities-debbie-jolly/
5. Welfare Reform Act *2012*: www.legislation.gov.uk/ukpga/2012/5/contents
6. Ellen Clifford, *The War on Disabled People* (Zed Books, 2020).
7. Michael Meacher, *Colin Traynor* (Hansard, 13 September 2012): https://hansard.parliament.uk/Commons/2012-09-13/debates/12091335000001/details
8. George Osborne, speech (*New Statesman*, October 2012): www.newstatesman.com/business/economics/2012/10/george-osbornes-speech-conservative-conference-full-text
9. Alison Little, 'Sick Benefits: 75% Are Faking' (*Express*, 27 July 2011): www.express.co.uk/news/uk/261337/Sick-benefits-75-are-faking
10. Amanda Williams, 'Workshy Map of Britain Revealed: Thousands of Incapacity Benefit Claimants Found to Be Capable of Working' (*Daily Mail*, 4 May 2013): www.dailymail.co.uk/news/article-2319355/Workshy-map-Britain-revealed-Thousands-incapacity-benefit-claimants-capable-working.html
11. John Pring, 'National Newspapers "Add Fuel to the Hate Crime Fire"' (Disability News Service, 3 September 2012): www.disabilitynewsservice.com/ministers-warned-over-adding-fuel-to-disablist-fire/

12. John Pring, 'Portraying Disabled People as "Parasites" Could Lead to "Violence and Killings", Says UN Chair' (Disability News Service, 14 September 2017): www.disabilitynewsservice.com/portraying-disabled-people-as-parasites-could-lead-to-violence-and-killings-says-un-chair/
13. Spartacus, 'The People's Review of the Work Capability Assessment' (Citizen Network, November 2012): https://citizen-network.org/uploads/attachment/409/the-peoples-review-of-the-wca.pdf
14. Malcolm Harrington, *Work Capability Assessment Independent Review – Year 3* (DWP, 20 November 2012): www.gov.uk/government/publications/work-capability-assessment-independent-review-year-3
15. *Atos Work Capability Assessments* (Hansard, 17 January 2013): https://hansard.parliament.uk/commons/2013-01-17/debates/13011761000001/AtosWorkCapabilityAssessments
16. David Cameron, 'Crazy Situation Where You Earn More on Benefits Than You Do at Work Ends NOW' (*Sun*, 6 April 2013): www.thesun.co.uk/archives/politics/649702/crazy-situation-where-you-earn-more-on-benefits-than-you-do-at-work-ends-now/
17. Sophie Hutchinson, 'Disability Benefit Assessments "Unfair", Says Ex-worker' (BBC, 16 May 2013): www.bbc.co.uk/news/uk-22546036
18. John Pring, 'DWP Declares "Business as Usual", Despite Appeal Court Ruling' (Disability News Service, 17 January 2014): www.disabilitynewsservice.com/dwp-declares-business-as-usual-despite-appeal-court-ruling/
19. China Mills and John Pring, 'Weaponising Time in the War on Welfare' (Critical Social Policy, 26 July 2023): https://journals.sagepub.com/doi/10.1177/02610183231187588

CHAPTER 12

1. Oral evidence, *Benefit Sanctions Policy beyond the Oakley Review* (Work and Pensions Committee, 4 February 2015): https://committees.parliament.uk/event/8332/formal-meeting-oral-evidence-session/
2. David Cameron (*The Andrew Marr Show*, BBC, 19 April 2015).
3. Gill Thompson, 'David Clapson: Sanctioned to Death?' (CrowdJustice, 2016): www.crowdjustice.com/case/david-clapson/

CHAPTER 13

1. Katriona Ormiston, 'Man Starved after Benefits Were Cut' (*Oxford Mail*, 28 February 2014): www.oxfordmail.co.uk/news/11043378.man-starved-benefits-cut/

2. Amelia Gentleman, 'Vulnerable Man Starved to Death after Benefits Were Cut' (*Guardian*, 28 February 2014): www.theguardian.com/society/2014/feb/28/man-starved-to-death-after-benefits-cut
3. Vicky Smith, 'Disabled Man Starved to Death after Benefits Cut When Atos Declared Him Fit for Work' (*Mirror*, 28 February 2014): www.mirror.co.uk/news/uk-news/disabled-mark-wood-starved-death-3194250

CHAPTER 14

1. John Pring, 'Criminal Justice Agencies Reject Call to Investigate Duncan Smith's WCA Failings' (Disability News Service, 22 December 2016): www.disabilitynewsservice.com/criminal-justice-agencies-reject-call-to-investigate-duncan-smiths-wca-failings/

CHAPTER 15

1. Toby Helm, 'Labour Will Be Tougher Than Tories on Benefits, Promises New Welfare Chief' (*Guardian*, 12 October 2013): www.theguardian.com/politics/2013/oct/12/labour-benefits-tories-labour-rachel-reeves-welfare
2. Press release, 'Benefit Sanctions – Ending the "Something for Nothing" Culture' (DWP, 6 November 2013): https://webarchive.nationalarchives.gov.uk/ukgwa/20131113073109/https:/www.gov.uk/government/news/benefit-sanctions-ending-the-something-for-nothing-culture
3. Dr Paul Litchfield, *An Independent Review of the Work Capability Assessment – Year Four* (DWP, December 2013): https://assets.publishing.service.gov.uk/government/uploads/system/uploads/attachment_data/file/265351/work-capability-assessment-year-4-paul-litchfield.pdf
4. Investigation report, *Who Benefits? The Benefits Assessment and Death of Ms DE* (Mental Welfare Commission for Scotland, March 2014): www.mwcscot.org.uk/sites/default/files/2019-06/who_benefits_final.pdf

CHAPTER 16

1. John Pring, 'Lib Dem Minister Casts Doubt on DWP Response on Benefits Deaths' (Disability News Service, 10 October 2014): www.disabilitynewsservice.com/lib-dem-minister-casts-doubt-on-dwp-response-on-benefits-deaths/
2. John Pring, 'Incompetence, Discrimination and "Fraud": The US Company That Could Take over from Atos' (Disability News Service,

17 October 2014): www.disabilitynewsservice.com/incompetence-discrimination-and-fraud-the-us-company-that-could-take-over-from-atos/

3. Dr Paul Litchfield, *An Independent Review of the Work Capability Assessment – Year Five* (DWP, November 2014): https://assets.publishing.service.gov.uk/government/uploads/system/uploads/attachment_data/file/380027/wca-fifth-independent-review.pdf

CHAPTER 17

1. *Regulation 28: Prevention of Future Deaths Report* (Courts and Tribunals Judiciary, 20 January 2016): www.judiciary.uk/wp-content/uploads/2022/06/Faiza-Ahmed-2016-0600_Redacted.pdf
2. Simon Hattenstone, 'Faiza Ahmed: How One Woman's Cries for Help Were Missed by Every Authority' (*Guardian*, 6 February 2016): www.theguardian.com/uk-news/2016/feb/06/faiza-ahmed-cries-for-help-missed-every-authority-simon-hattenstone

CHAPTER 18

1. *Regulation 28: Prevention of Future Deaths Report* (Courts and Tribunals Judiciary, 13 January 2014): www.judiciary.uk/wp-content/uploads/2014/06/OSullivan-2014-0012.pdf
2. John Pring, 'Coroner's "Ground-breaking" Verdict: Suicide Was "Triggered" by "Fit for Work" Test' (Disability News Service, 18 September 2015): www.disabilitynewsservice.com/coroners-ground-breaking-verdict-suicide-was-triggered-by-fit-for-work-test/
3. John Pring, 'Activist Felt "Violated" after Judge Used Google to Compile Dossier' (Disability News Service, 13 March 2015): www.disabilitynewsservice.com/activist-felt-violated-after-judge-used-google-to-compile-dossier/
4. 'DWP Panic and Cover-up after Claimant Death Publicity' (Benefits and Work, 13 September 2016): www.benefitsandwork.co.uk/news/dwp-panic-and-cover-up-after-claimant-death-publicity-wca-medics-warned-we-cannot-defend-you
5. Angus Robertson, *Prime Minister's Questions* (Hansard, 21 October 2015): https://hansard.parliament.uk/commons/2015-10-21/debates/15102145000036/Engagements#contribution-15102145000158
6. Iain Duncan Smith, 'Anger over IDS "Work Your Way out of Poverty" Call' (Disability News Service, 9 October 2015): www.

disabilitynewsservice.com/tory-conference-anger-over-ids-work-your-way-out-of-poverty-call/

CHAPTER 19

1. Ben Barr et al., '"First, Do No Harm": Are Disability Assessments Associated with Adverse Trends in Mental Health?' (*Journal of Epidemiology and Community Health*, November 2015): https://jech.bmj.com/content/70/4/339
2. Deaths by Welfare podcast, *Zero Points: The Work Capability Assessment* (Healing Justice Ldn, May 2023): https://healingjusticeldn.org/resources/dwp-ep4/
3. Welfare Reform and Work Act 2016: www.legislation.gov.uk/ukpga/2016/7/contents/enacted/data.htm
4. John Pring, 'DWP Issued Guidance That Made Suicides More Likely, Then "Lied" to Cover Its Tracks' (Disability News Service, 29 September 2016): www.disabilitynewsservice.com/dwp-issued-guidance-that-made-suicides-more-likely-then-lied-to-cover-its-tracks/
5. 'ESA: Outcomes of Work Capability Assessments Including Mandatory Reconsiderations and Appeals' (DWP, 8 September 2016): www.gov.uk/government/statistics/esa-outcomes-of-work-capability-assessments-including-mandatory-reconsiderations-and-appeals-september-2016
6. 'DWP FOI Releases for May 2016' (DWP, 12 May 2016): www.gov.uk/government/publications/dwp-foi-releases-for-may-2016
7. *Inquiry Report* (UN Committee on the Rights of Persons with Disabilities, 2 September 2016): https://tbinternet.ohchr.org/_layouts/15/TreatyBodyExternal/TBSearch.aspx?Lang=en&TreatyID=4&DocTypeCategoryID=7
8. Patrick Butler, 'Damian Green Dismisses "Offensive" UN Report on UK Disability Rights' (*Guardian*, 8 November 2016): www.theguardian.com/society/2016/nov/08/damian-green-dismisses-offensive-un-report-on-uk-disability-rights
9. John Pring, 'Information Commissioner Questions DWP's "Highly Unusual" Failure on Benefit Deaths' (Disability News Service, 2 March 2017): www.disabilitynewsservice.com/information-commissioner-questions-dwps-highly-unusual-failure-on-benefit-deaths/

CHAPTER 20

1. John Pring, '"Staggering" ESA Suicide Figures Prompt Calls for Inquiry and Prosecution of Ministers' (Disability News Service, 14 December

2017): www.disabilitynewsservice.com/staggering-esa-suicide-figures-prompt-calls-for-inquiry-and-prosecution-of-ministers/

2. Petition, *Justice for Jodey Whiting. Independent Inquiry into Deaths Linked to the DWP* (UK Parliament, March 2019): https://petition.parliament.uk/archived/petitions/243337
3. Dr Paul Williams, *Prime Minister's Questions* (Hansard, 13 March 2019): https://hansard.parliament.uk/commons/2019-03-13/debates/5F2B8816-2B09-4EDB-9AC6-0A5C6CFE3876/Engagements#contribution-1F54FBA7-5F42-4DB8-91E7-FAD6308BD7EA
4. Joy Dove with Ann and Joe Cusack, *A Mother's Job* (Mirror Books, 13 October 2022): https://blackwells.co.uk/bookshop/product/A-Mothers-Job-by-Joy-Dove-Ann-Cusack-Joe-Cusack/9781915306159
5. *Joy Dove vs HM Assistant Coroner for Teesside and Hartlepool and Dr Shareen Rahman* (Court of Appeal (Civil Division), 17 March 2023): www.bailii.org/ew/cases/EWCA/Civ/2023/289.html
6. 'Coroner Promises "Full and Fearless" Second Inquest into Death of Jodey Whiting' (Leigh Day, 24 November 2023): www.leighday.co.uk/news/news/2023-news/coroner-promises-full-and-fearless-second-inquest-into-death-of-jodey-whiting/

CHAPTER 21

1. Benjamin Kentish, 'Government Cuts Have Caused "Human Catastrophe" for Disabled, UN Committee Says' (*Independent*, 25 August 2017): www.independent.co.uk/news/uk/politics/government-spending-cuts-human-catastrophe-un-committee-rights-persons-with-disabilities-disabled-people-a7911556.html
2. John Pring, 'PIP Investigation: 200 Cases of Dishonesty… and Still DWP, Atos and Capita Refuse to Act' (Disability News Service, 3 August 2017): www.disabilitynewsservice.com/pip-investigation-200-cases-of-dishonesty-and-still-dwp-atos-and-capita-refuse-to-act/
3. Steve Griffiths, 'Dark Times for Those That Cannot Work' (Compass, October 2010).
4. Dave Smith, *Stop Private Contracting out of Health-Related Assessments for DWP Benefits* (UK Parliament, 2019): https://petition.parliament.uk/archived/petitions/274312
5. *Tribunal Statistics Quarterly: April to June 2019* (Ministry of Justice, 12 September 2019): www.gov.uk/government/statistics/tribunal-statistics-quarterly-april-to-june-2019
6. *Personal Independence Payment Claimant Research* (DWP, September 2018): https://assets.publishing.service.gov.uk/government/uploads/

system/uploads/attachment_data/file/738909/summary-personal-independence-payment-claimant-research-final-report.pdf

CHAPTER 22

1. *Safeguarding Adults Review* (Nottingham City Safeguarding Adults Board, May 2023):https://www.nottinghamcity.gov.uk/media/xrpcivn3/sar-valentina-final-for-publication-may-2023.pdf

CHAPTER 23

1. Danny Taggart, Ellen Clifford et al., '"They Say Jump, We Say How High?" Conditionality, Sanctioning and Incentivising Disabled People into the UK Labour Market' (Disability and Society, May 2020): www.tandfonline.com/doi/abs/10.1080/09687599.2020.1766422?journalCode=cdso20
2. Oral evidence: *Health Assessments for Benefits* (Work and Pensions Committee, 1 December 2021): https://committees.parliament.uk/oralevidence/3121/pdf/
3. John Pring, 'DWP Secretly Abandons Work on £100m Plan to Prevent Suicides and Learn from Errors' (Disability News Service, 8 December 2022): www.disabilitynewsservice.com/dwp-secretly-abandons-work-on-100m-plan-to-prevent-suicides-and-learn-from-errors/
4. John Pring, 'Coffey Scrapped Plan for Independent Review of Sanctions, DWP Admits' (Disability News Service, 26 January 2023): www.disabilitynewsservice.com/coffey-scrapped-plan-for-independent-review-of-sanctions-dwp-admits/
5. *Information Held by the Department for Work and Pensions on Deaths by Suicide of Benefit Claimants* (National Audit Office, 7 February 2020): www.nao.org.uk/reports/information-held-by-the-department-for-work-pensions-on-deaths-by-suicide-of-benefit-claimants/
6. *Alison Turner vs secretary of state for work and pensions* (High Court, 3 March 2021): www.bailii.org/ew/cases/EWHC/Admin/2021/465.html
7. *Safeguarding Adults Review* (Nottingham City Safeguarding Adults Board, May 2023): www.nottinghamcity.gov.uk/information-for-residents/health-and-social-care/adult-social-care/adult-safeguarding/safeguarding-adults-reviews/

CHAPTER 24

1. Richard Butchins, *The Truth about Disability Benefits* (Channel 4 *Dispatches*, 17 December 2021): www.channel4.com/programmes/truth-about-disability-benefits-dispatches

2. John Pring, 'Partner of "Distraught" ESA Claimant Says DWP Drove Him to His Death' (Disability News Service, 4 February 2021): www.disabilitynewsservice.com/partner-of-distraught-esa-claimant-says-dwp-drove-him-to-his-death/
3. John Pring, 'DWP Hounded Disabled Woman for Years before Her "Starvation" Death, Papers Show' (Disability News Service, 8 September 2022): www.disabilitynewsservice.com/dwp-hounded-disabled-woman-for-years-before-her-starvation-death-papers-show/
4. John Pring, 'PIP Claimant Took His Own Life after Paramedic "Ignored His Pain" and DWP Cut His Benefits' (Disability News Service, 27 February 2020): www.disabilitynewsservice.com/pip-claimant-took-his-own-life-after-paramedic-ignored-his-pain-and-dwp-cut-his-benefits/
5. Mel Stride, *Letter to Sir Stephen Timms* (Commons Work and Pensions Committee, 25 October 2023): https://committees.parliament.uk/work/7866/safeguarding-vulnerable-claimants/publications/3/correspondence/
6. John Pring, 'DWP Admits Court Defeat after Universal Credit Discrimination Led to Suicide Thoughts' (Disability News Service, 27 October 2022): www.disabilitynewsservice.com/dwp-admits-court-defeat-after-universal-credit-discrimination-led-to-suicide-thoughts/
7. *Deaths by Welfare Project* (Healing Justice Ldn): https://healingjusticeldn.org/deaths-by-welfare-project/
8. Jamie Redman and Del Fletcher, 'Violent Bureaucracy: A Critical Analysis of the British Public Employment Service' (Critical Social Policy, January 2021): http://shura.shu.ac.uk/28060/
9. John Pring, 'DWP Apologises to Autistic Man after Work Coach Threatens to Stick Pins in His Eyes' (Disability News Service, 2 December 2021): www.disabilitynewsservice.com/dwp-apologises-to-autistic-man-after-work-coach-threatens-to-stick-pins-in-his-eyes/
10. Kirsty Gomersal, *Kevin Gale: Prevention of Future Deaths Report* (Courts and Tribunals Judiciary, 8 November 2023): www.judiciary.uk/prevention-of-future-death-reports/kevin-gale-prevention-of-future-deaths-report/

EPILOGUE

1. *Transforming Support: The Health and Disability White Paper* (DWP, 15 March 2023): www.gov.uk/government/publications/transforming-support-the-health-and-disability-white-paper

2. 'Staffing Crisis in the DWP' (PCS, December 2023): https://mypcs.my.salesforce.com/sfc/p/#1t0000000ksc/a/Sl00001RxIo/bhm_vagoggsLocvkItbfXZEbpNh7dQ7cNxqPBj.vOA8
3. *Consultation Outcome: Work Capability Assessment: Activities and Descriptors* (DWP, 22 November 2023): www.gov.uk/government/consultations/work-capability-assessment-activities-and-descriptors
4. *Economic and Fiscal Outlook* (Office for Budget Responsibility, November 2023): https://obr.uk/docs/dlm_uploads/E03004355_November-Economic-and-Fiscal-Outlook_Web-Accessible.pdf
5. Carol Monaghan, *PACE Trial: People with ME* (Hansard, 20 February 2018): https://hansard.parliament.uk/Commons/2018-02-20/debates/990746C7-9010-4566-940D-249F5026FF73/PACETrialPeopleWithME
6. Vickie Cooper and David Whyte (eds), *The Violence of Austerity* (Pluto Press, 2017).
7. Sue Jones, 'The "Still Face" Paradigm and the Department for Work and Pensions' (Politics and Insights, February 2023): https://politicsandinsights.org/2023/02/23/the-still-face-paradigm-and-the-department-for-work-and-pensions/
8. Sue Jones, 'The Still Face Paradigm, the Just World Fallacy, Inequality and the Decline of Empathy' (Politics and Insights, January 2017): https://politicsandinsights.org/2017/01/09/still-face-paradigm-the-just-world-fallacy-and-the-decline-of-empathy/
9. John Pring, 'Broadcaster's Silence over "Rabblerouser" Tweet on Disability Benefits' (Disability News Service, 1 June 2023): www.disabilitynewsservice.com/broadcasters-silence-over-rabblerouser-tweet-on-disability-benefits/
10. Alex Clark and Tom Haynes, 'Exactly How Much of Your Salary Goes towards Britain's Growing Welfare State' (*Telegraph*, 12 June 2023): www.telegraph.co.uk/money/tax/news/britain-working-costing-calculate-pay-benefits-tax/
11. John Pring, 'Disability Minister Faces Resignation Calls after Posting "Dangerous" and Hostile Video' (Disability News Service, 27 April 2023): www.disabilitynewsservice.com/disability-minister-faces-resignation-calls-after-posting-dangerous-and-hostile-video/
12. China Mills and John Pring, 'Weaponising Time in the War on Welfare' (*Critical Social Policy*, July 2023): https://journals.sagepub.com/doi/10.1177/02610183231187588

Index of pages that could be triggering, and summary of subject matter

Index